Beauty Therapy
The Basics

Maxine Whittaker, Debbie Forsythe-Conroy and Judith Ifould

Hodder & Stoughton

A MEMBER OF THE HODDER HEADLINE GROUP

D0183991

Orders: please contact Bookpoint Ltd, 39 Milton Park, Abingdon, Oxon OX14 4TD. Telephone: (44) 01235 400414, Fax: (44) 01235 400454. Lines are open from 9.00–6.00, Monday to Saturday, with a 24 hour message answering service. Email address: orders@bookpoint.co.uk

British Library Cataloguing in Publication Data
A catalogue record for this title is available from The British Library

ISBN 0 340 730730

First published 1999
Impression number   10 9 8 7 6 5 4 3
Year   2005 2004 2003 2002 2001 2000

Typeset by Wearset, Boldon, Tyne and Wear.
Printed in Italy for Hodder & Stoughton Educational, a division of Hodder Headline Plc, 338 Euston Road, London NW1 3BH by Printer Trento.

Contents

Preface

This book has been written in line with the new Standards for SVQ/NVQ in Beauty Therapy at level 2 and as far as possible the language and format follows those Standards.

The book will provide the necessary essential knowledge and understanding to meet the requirements of the Standards with further reading sections providing the student with the opportunity to study some topics in more depth.

There are tasks within each chapter which have been designed to generate appropriate supplementary evidence for a student's portfolio as well as review questions at the end of each chapter for students to review their own learning.

With the increasing demand for key skills to be accredited, we have written key skills tasks which will help to identify assessment opportunities within the beauty therapy salon for key skills. Whilst every effort to cross reference these tasks with the NVQ key skills criteria has been made, it has not been possible to identify specific levels because of the needs of different qualifications (eg the new Modern Apprenticeship scheme for Beauty Therapy). The tasks should therefore be used as examples which can be expanded upon to meet the requirements of different levels and different assessment situations as required.

We have endeavoured to put together a book which will support students and trainees as well as tutors and trainers in their learning and teaching. We hope that *Beauty Therapy – The Basics for NVQ Level 2* provides an invaluable source of practical and theoretical information to suport learning whether in the salon, college or training school.

Acknowledgements

I would like to thank my colleagues from De Montfort University for the years of work we undertook together as a team to develop NVQs in Beauty Therapy.

Their dedication to the NVQ philosophy in providing access to beauty therapy education and training for a much wider range of individuals and their hard work in adapting learning and assessment materials to meet the needs of their students and competence based assessment has inspired me to write material for this book.

Thanks in particular to Kirsty Wych for sharing her experience in delivering and assessing key skills and to Vicki Baldwin a Sugaring Practitioner for providing me with extra information on sugaring methods of hair removal.

Thanks to City & Guilds for their support and co-operation in providing up to date information on The Standards and objective reading of our work.

Finally my thanks must go to my husband, Roger, for his encouragement, patience and his tolerance as the work for the book disrupted our lives as he coped with endless paper, my constant word processing and my very short temper!

Maxine Whittaker

I would like to thank my colleagues at Bradford and Ilkley Community College for their inspiration, dedication and enthusiasm to Beauty Therapy. I would also like to thank my husband Chris for his encouragement and support. Finally, I would like to thank my son Alex for providing me with the motivation to contribute to this book. I promise to make up for the lost weekends!

Debbie Forsythe-Conroy

The publishers would like to thank Jackie Cox, Head of the School of Hairdressing and Beauty Therapy at Basingstoke College of Technology, who gave permission for photos to be taken; Gary Roberts for the photos taken at Basingstoke and Judith Ifould for photos of nail conditions. Ellison's provided the photo on page 290.

Introduction

Beauty therapy is a fast growing industry with employment opportunities in beauty therapy salons, health spas, cosmetic houses, cruise ships and working abroad. Training to a high standard is essential to enable you to access these opportunities anywhere in the United Kingdom or abroad.

National Vocational Qualifications (NVQs) are designed to assess a student's ability to do a particular job according to standards set by employers in that industry. In other words, when you have successfully completed an NVQ and apply for a job the employer will immediately know what you are capable of doing. There are other qualifications in beauty therapy besides the NVQ which are recognised by the beauty therapy industry. The information contained in this book will meet the needs of all students of beauty therapy regardless of which qualification they are working towards.

NVQs are based on assessment of **practical skills**, **knowledge** and **understanding** at levels 1, 2, 3 or 4. Broadly speaking, level 1 is an introduction to beauty therapy – you might be an assistant helping therapists in a salon. Level 2 includes using various practical skills to treat clients in the salon. Level 3 involves learning more complex treatments as well as supervising staff. Level 4 is management training for the qualified and experienced therapist.

The qualification is made up of **Units** which describe a particular treatment or job within the salon. Each unit is made up of several Elements containing **Performance Criteria (PCs)**, range statements and underpinning knowledge. The awarding body will provide you with an assessment log book which contains all the detail you require to cover the National Standards.

Before assessment can take place you must be familiar with the requirements of each unit and undertake practical and theoretical instruction either in the workplace or at a recognised training centre such as a college of further education. Your lecturer will provide learning opportunities through demonstrations followed by practice on clients in the salon, as well as theory lessons to provide you with the necessary underpinning knowledge and understanding.

Assessment for an NVQ is based on you, the candidate, being able to demonstrate that you can do the job. Your skills are measured against the National Standards by a qualified assessor who is trained to make judgements about your ability.

The assessor will usually be your lecturer who will make sure that you are able to carry out treatments safely and competently before assessing you. Your assessor will advise you on assessment opportunities: observation of practical work, oral questioning, written tests, case studies and assignments. You will also compile a **portfolio**. The assessor will discuss the assessment criteria with you before an assessment takes place and agree how the assessment will be carried out. This will usually involve your assessor watching you work. This is called assessment by **observation**. The assessor will need to be sure that you understand what you are doing and why. This will involve asking you questions. This is called **oral questioning**. As most of your work involves a client this will usually be done after your client has left, unless the assessor wishes to confirm something with you during the treatment.

Portfolio evidence requires you to collect materials together to confirm your skills and demonstrate your understanding. This type of evidence can be divided into **performance evidence** and **knowledge evidence**. Performance evidence includes items such as client record cards, photographs, case studies witness testimonies which help to confirm that you can carry out a task. Knowledge evidence will be such things as written tests and assignments which show that you have gained knowledge of a subject.

These items are usually collected together in a portfolio (a file or folder), to form part of the assessment for each unit. You are required to provide a guide for your assessor so that the information contained in your portfolio is organised. This is called **referencing**.

Verification is a process to ensure that assessment is fair. It involves someone who is trained to observe assessments taking place and who looks at assignments and written tests. The **internal verifier** will check that the assessment processes are fair and valid and sign off your assessment log book, before claiming certification from the awarding body. The training centre will retain your portfolio and assessment log book for the **external verifier** who does a further check on behalf of the awarding body.

This book has been written to help you with all aspects of NVQ **level 2 beauty therapy**. Each unit follows the units of the National Standards and uses the same headings for ease of reference. Each unit contains sections covering:

- knowledge requirements
- activities, some of which can be used to generate evidence for your portfolio
- self assessment tasks to test knowledge and understanding
- key skills tasks which will help to provide evidence for assessment against the Key Skills Standards.

UNIT 1

Support the health, safety and security of the salon environment

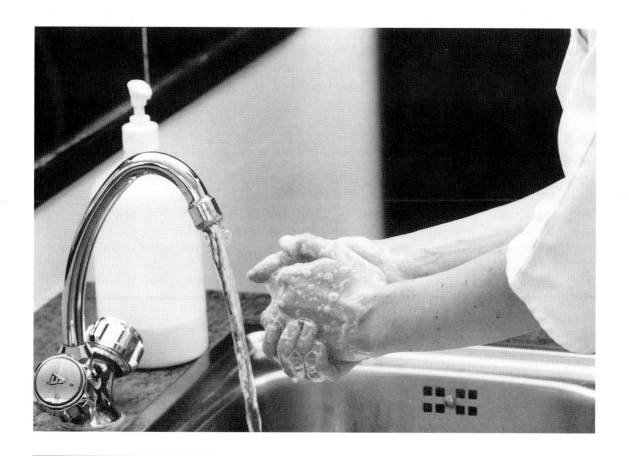

In this unit you will learn about:

- health and safety in the salon
- the laws relating to beauty therapy practice
- emergency procedures
- personal presentation and salon hygiene procedures
- safe salon working practices
- salon rules and regulations
- hazards in the salon
- safe working conditions.

INTRODUCTION

The work place can hold many dangers and it is everyone's responsibility to ensure that the salon is a safe and hygienic environment. The beauty therapist has additional responsibilities when working with clients. There is a **legal requirement** to ensure that the general public are not at risk when visiting the salon and receiving treatment.

THE LAW RELATING TO BEAUTY THERAPY PRACTICE

Health and Safety at Work Act 1974

This is the main Act of Parliament governing the duties and responsibilities of employers and employees whilst at work. The Health and Safety at Work Act (HASAW) is an 'enabling' Act which covers a whole range of legislation relating to health and safety.

The duties of the employer

The employer must:

- manage and promote safe working practices in the work place
- provide a healthy environment through clean, tidy, well lit and ventilated work areas
- ensure employees are adequately qualified and to provide training as necessary.

If there are more than five employees a written **Health and Safety Policy** is required.

The duties of the employee

The employee must:

- follow salon rules and regulations
- cooperate with the employer in all matters of health and safety
- follow safe working practices and attend training as required.

All individuals have responsibility for health and safety whilst at work.

The findings of the **Health and Safety Executive** and the demands of **European legislation** have lead to a number of new laws. These are discussed in the following pages.

The Electricity at Work Regulations 1992

The beauty therapist uses a range of electrical equipment which must be tested by a qualified electrician at least once a year. A sticker will usually be placed on each item giving the date it was tested. If not, a record of equipment inspection and servicing must be available on request.

When using any electrical equipment you should make the following checks:
- Equipment should not be used near basins or where liquids are likely to be spilt on the appliance.
- Cables, flexes, connections, sockets and plugs must be intact with no exposed wiring.
- The appliance should be on a level and stable trolley.
- The appliance must be switched off and disconnected from the mains when not in use.
- Cables and flexes must not be allowed to trail across the floor as they could cause someone to trip.
- Electrical equipment should be stored carefully by winding flexes and cables smoothly round the appliance.
- At the end of the working day someone must take the responsibility to check that all appliances are switched off and disconnected.

> **NOTE!** Remember not to touch sockets, connections, plugs or wires with damp or wet hands. If you come across faulty or damaged electrical equipment take it out of use immediately by placing a clearly written 'out of order sign' on it. Report the fault to the manager.

Wiring a plug

It is important that all relevant staff make visual safety checks and understand the wiring of a plug.

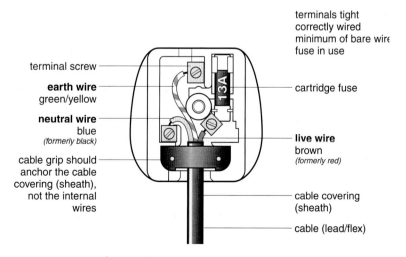

terminals tight
correctly wired
minimum of bare wire
fuse in use

terminal screw

earth wire
green/yellow

neutral wire
blue
(formerly black)

cable grip should
anchor the cable
covering (sheath),
not the internal
wires

13A

cartridge fuse

live wire
brown
(formerly red)

cable covering
(sheath)

cable (lead/flex)

Figure 1.1 All salon staff should understand the wiring of a plug

The Personal Protective Equipment at Work Regulations 1992

This legislation places a requirement on the employer to:

- provide suitable and sufficient protective clothing and equipment for all employees, eg rubber gloves
- ensure that equipment is suitable for its purpose and kept in good repair
- that staff have been adequately trained in the use of chemicals and equipment.

Workplace (Health, Safety and Welfare) Regulations 1992

These regulations have taken the place of most of the **Office Shops and Railway Premises Act 1963** and deal with the working environment, heating, lighting, ventilation, cleanliness and rest room facilities and the maintenance of a safe and healthy working environment.

Control of Substances Hazardous to Health Regulations 1988 (COSHH)

The employer is required to regulate employees' exposure to substances which may cause ill health or injury. The potential risks to all those working in the salon are assessed. This process is called **risk assessment** and is normally carried out by the salon manager.

Risk assessment

Risk assessment involves making a list of all the substances used in the salon or sold to clients which may be hazardous to health, because they may:

- cause irritation
- burn the skin
- give off fumes
- cause allergic reactions.

Instructions for handling and disposal of these substances are then made available to all staff with training if required. Manufacturers will normally supply information relating to their products.

Hazard warning symbols

These symbols appear on packaging and labels (see Figure 1.3).

The Manual Handling Operations Regulations 1992

These regulations require everyone in the work place to minimise risks from lifting and handling large or heavy objects. The beauty therapist must take particular care when moving equipment in the salon (see Figure 1.4).

Equipment should be fixed on a suitable trolley and free standing equipment should be on castors for ease of movement around the salon. Trolleys must be checked regularly to ensure that

	Specification	Health hazard	Use/handling	Storage	Disposal	Caution/action
Fine powders	Surface cleaners Nail dry sprays Hairsprays	Flammable	Do not smoke. Keep away from eyes. Use in well ventilated areas	Cool dry place. Avoid sunlight. Avoid excessive temperatures	Do not pierce or burn container (explosive)	In case of fire evacuate areas known to contain aerosols
Caustic	Cuticle remover	Substances which can burn the skin	Keep away from eyes. Do not use on sensitive skin	Cool dry place	Wear gloves. Mop up spills with damp cloth (rinse well)	Eye/skin contact – wash area and seek medical advice. Indigestion – drink plenty of water
Flammable	Surgical spirit Acetone Astringent Eau de cologne Equipment cleaner Flowers of sulphur Nail polish thinners Nail polish remover Rose water Solvents Witchazel	Flammable vapours	Do not smoke. Label clearly. Good ventilation	Distinguish inflammables from flammables. Store in cool place keep sealed	Seek advice from EHO	Wask skin or eyes immediately. Remove to fresh air if inhaled, then seek medication
Sensitising	Equipment cleaner Gluteral dehyde solution Acrylic nail powder Resin gel Nail glue Nail off remover Nail primer Lash tint	May cause allergic reaction	Wear gloves	Cool dry place	Use normal disposal methods or contact EHO for large amounts	Eye/skin contact. Wash immediately. Inhalation – move to fresh air. Indigestion – seek medical advice
Skin bleach	All bleach products Hydrogen peroxide	May cause skin irritation	Wear gloves. Avoid inhalation	Cool dry place	Do not incinerate. Dilute to mop up spillage. Wash powders down drains	Eye/skin contact – wash immediately. Inhalation – remove to fresh air, then seek medical advice
Fine powders	Acrylic nail powder Bleaches Bronzing powder Calamine powder Face powder Flowers of sulphur Fullers earth Kaolin Magnesium carbonate	Inhalation can cause irritation	Avoid inhalation	Cool dry place. Closed container	Treat as domestic waste. (Flowers of sulphur is a fire hazard)	Eye/skin contact – rinse immediately with water, do not inhale
Contaminated sharps	Needles/blades etc	Cross infection risk	Used items should be placed in sharps containers	Secure storage	Consult EHO. Can be incinerated at local hospital	Seek medical attention

EHO – Environmental Health Officer

Figure 1.2 Table of major chemical hazards

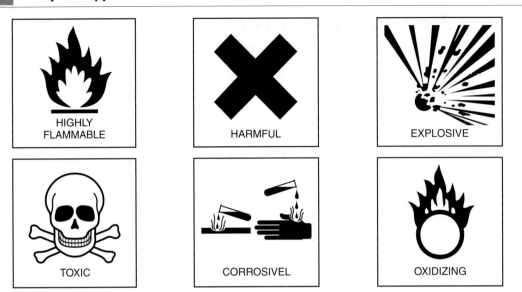

Figure 1.3 You should be familiar with hazard warning symbols

they are stable and that the castors run freely. However, equipment should not be moved unnecessarily in particular equipment containing hot liquids such as wax.

Lifting

Good posture and correct lifting techniques must be followed to avoid injury.

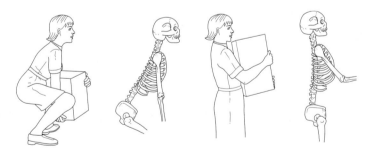

Figure 1.4 Learn how to lift correctly, so that you do not strain your back

The Fire Precautions Act 1971

This is concerned with fire prevention and adequate means of escape in the event of a fire. The employer must apply for a **fire certificate** if the business employs 20 or more staff and follow strict regulations on fire prevention.

Fire precautions are essential in all business premises and involve ensuring that:
- fire escapes are kept free of obstruction, are clearly sign posted and doors can be opened easily
- all employees are made aware of evacuation procedures for the salon and that there is regular fire drill practice
- fire-fighting equipment suitable for all types of fire is easily reached and kept in good working order
- all staff are familiar with the salon's emergency procedures and use of fire-fighting equipment
- smoke alarms are fitted
- fire doors are fitted to help control the spread of fire.

Fire extinguishers

Different fire extinguishers are made to deal with different types of fire. From 1997, all fire extinguishers in the UK must be coloured red and use symbols to show what type of fire they can be used for. It is vital that you use the right extinguisher for the fire type.

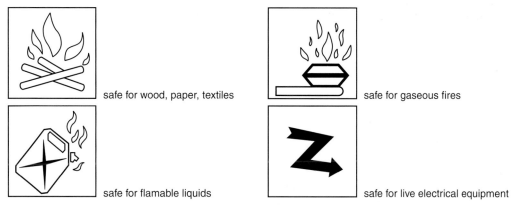

safe for wood, paper, textiles

safe for gaseous fires

safe for flamable liquids

safe for live electrical equipment

Figure 1.5 These symbols show which fire extinguishers can be used on different types of fire

The Local Government (Miscellaneous Provisions) Act 1982 (Local Authority Licensing)

The beauty therapist carries out some treatments such as ear piercing, micro-pigmentation, waxing, eyebrow shaping and electrical epilation which require particular attention to hygiene. This is due to the increased risk of cross infection from blood or body fluids coming into contact with the therapist, equipment or other clients.

Guidelines are available from the **Local Authority** and under the local bylaws inspection of the premises to check hygiene procedures will be necessary. When the Environmental Health Inspector (EHO) is satisfied that the premises are of the required standard, the business will become registered and receive a certificate. An inspector will pay particular attention to:

- cleaning and sterilising of implements
- safe working practices with materials such as disposable needles
- salon cleaning to a high standard
- therapists' personal hygiene and working practices.

Activity

Working in a small group, write to your local authority requesting information on the local bylaws relating to the beauty therapy salon. You may find that different Local Authorities send different information and have slightly different regulations. This is because bylaws are based on local needs and the interpretation of government guide-lines may vary to meet these needs.

The Reporting of Injuries, Diseases and Dangerous Occurrences Regulations 1985 (RIDDOR)

These regulations ensure that any incident occurring in the work place and leading to an injury or a condition resulting from a work activity is recorded in an **accident book**.

INSPECTION AND REGISTRATION

All businesses must comply with the law on health and safety. To ensure that this happens the **Environmental Health Department** of the Local Authority will appoint an environmental health officer to visit and inspect the premises.

This inspector has the authority to demand that any hazards identified during the inspection are dealt with by the employer within a given period of time. This is called an **improvement notice**. Should the employer not comply with the notice by removing the danger within a given period of time, closure of the business can result, with the Local Authority issuing a **prohibition notice**.

INSURANCE

Whilst every effort must be made to prevent injury and disease it may be that unforeseen circumstances will lead to accidents in the work place. It is essential therefore that employers are covered by **insurance**.

The Employers Liability (Compulsory Insurance) Act 1969

The law requires the employer to provide insurance cover against claims for injury or illness as a result of negligence by the employer or other employees. The **certificate of insurance** must be displayed in the work place.

Public Liability Insurance

The employer is not required by law to take out insurance to cover claims from the public, but is well advised to do so. It is becoming increasingly common for clients to sue businesses for damages.

WHAT HEALTH AND SAFETY RISKS ARE THERE IN THE SALON?

The beauty therapy salon carries risks relating to the use of chemicals and electrical equipment as well as those of falling, fire, infection, scalds, burns and cuts.

Activity

Look around the salon you are working in and make a list of the hazards which could put you or your clients at risk of injury. (A list of likely hazards appears at the end of this unit on page 30 – cross check with our list.)

SELF ASSESSMENT TEST

1. The Act which covers the work place environment (heating, ventilation, rest room facilities) is:
    a) Control of Substances Hazardous to Health
    b) Local Government (Miscellaneous Provisions) Act
    c) Workplace (Health, Safety and Welfare) Regulations
    d) Personal Protective Equipment at Work regulations.
2. The Electricity at Work Regulations require the beauty therapist to:
    a) ensure that all electrical equipment in the salon is in safe working order
    b) switch on electrical heaters at the start of the day
    c) wear rubber gloves
    d) know the symbols on fire extinguishers.
3. If a beauty therapy salon does not follow health and safety regulations the Local Authority can close the salon down. This is called:

a) a property notice
b) an improvement notice
c) a health notice
d) a prohibition notice.

4. When making a visual safety check of electrical equipment before switching a machine on you must look at:
   a) the manufacturer's instructions
   b) the cables and flexes to check for frayed or worn areas where wires are exposed
   c) the red indicator light which tells you the machine is switched on
   d) the underneath of the machine.

5. When wiring a plug the live wire is always coloured:
   a) blue
   b) red
   c) brown
   d) green.

6. The hazard warning symbol for a toxic substance is:
   a) skull and cross bones
   b) a cross
   c) a flame
   d) a red band.

Element 1.1

Follow emergency procedures

All the staff must be prepared for emergency situations which may occur in the salon. Each person must take responsibility for the correct procedure to be carried out promptly and without panic. This can only be achieved by ensuring that everyone understands their role in an emergency and is trained to carry it out effectively. Individual members of staff should be identified as key people to handle an emergency: trained first aider, health and safety manager.

Staff training in health and safety is the responsibility of the salon owner or manager and should include:
- safe systems of work
- fire prevention
- risks and hazards found in the salon

- fire evacuation procedures
- emergency procedure in the event of an accident
- first aid.

FIRE

The risk of fire in the salon

The amount of **electrical equipment** used in the salon increases the risk of electrical fire. Over-loading electrical circuits or not following electrical safety procedures (eg ignoring worn cables) are the most common cause of electrical fires. Switch all equipment off at the mains immediately after use.

Chemicals which are flammable such as nail varnish remover and surgical spirit are a fire hazard and must be handled and stored in accordance with COSHH regulations (see page 5).

Depilitory wax and paraffin wax, if over heated, will give off fumes and may ignite. Thermostatically controlled heaters must be used and maintained regularly. Never leave heated wax unattended and do not carry heated wax from cubicle to cubicle.

Fires may be started by carelessness and poor working practices (ie drying towels over electrical or gas heaters, leaving appliances left switched on, discarding cigarettes). A **no smoking policy** should be in force in the salon to reduce the risk of fire.

Fire prevention

- The salon should be fitted with smoke alarms.
- Fire-fighting equipment must be available and located in an easily accessible area.
- Staff should know how to use the fire-fighting equipment and be able to identify the correct type of extinguisher to use on a particular fire.
- Safe working practices must be followed at all times.
- A no smoking policy should be in force.

Fire evacuation procedure

1. Each business premises should have an evacuation procedure which takes account of the emergency exit routes and fire escapes from the building.
2. Make sure you know where fire-fighting equipment is kept and how to use it.
3. You must take responsibility for your clients, who may be receiving treatment in different parts of the salon. Direct them to the nearest safe exit.
4. Switch off electrical equipment close by you at the mains.
5. Ensure that everyone has left the premises and congregated well away from the building.
6. If the fire is small and can be safely tackled with a fire extinguisher this can be carried out. However, you should not take any risks and the premises must be vacated quickly, closing as many doors as possible.

7. At the earliest possible time, the Emergency Services should be contacted by dialling 999 (see below). Give the exact address and details of the emergency.
8. Not all emergencies are caused by fires. Bomb scares are becoming more common with the need to evacuate a premises as quickly as possible, to get well away from the building and to follow police instructions.
9. Toxic fumes or gas leaks may also require evacuation from the building.
10. The salon should have regular emergency evacuation practice to familiarise staff with the procedure.

Activity

Check the emergency procedure for your salon and identify your role if a fire breaks out.

ACCIDENTS

Emergency procedures in the event of an accident
Calling the emergency services

1. Dial 999 (check whether your phone line requires an additional number to get an outside line).
2. Speak clearly stating what the emergency is and where you are.
3. Listen carefully to any instructions you are given.
4. Return to a safe place or to the patient.

Accidents in the workplace are often the result of unsafe working conditions or poor working practices. Staff may carry out treatments incorrectly or take unnecessary risks through lack of knowledge or training.

Any accident which occurs in the salon must be recorded in an **accident book**. If the accident is serious or if there are incidents of disease in the salon, **a report form** must be completed and sent to the Local Licensing Authority (see information on RIDDOR, page 8). These forms are more detailed than an accident book but fortunately are rarely required. The senior member of staff or the health and safety representative for the salon must be kept informed and take responsibility for the correct procedures being carried out.

The accident book

Keeping a record of all accidents, no matter how small, is essential. The entry in the accident book should be completed as soon as possible by a member of staff who saw the accident and can give an accurate account of what happened.

Details noted in the accident book should include:
- date
- time of the accident

- place where the accident occurred
- personal details of those involved – names, whether staff or client, contact details
- a brief description of what happened and the resulting injury
- what first aid was given
- whether the emergency services were called or the person(s) taken to hospital. If so, it is likely that the accident would be regarded as serious and an incident report form would also be required.

Activity

Ask to see the accident book in your salon. Note the types of accidents recorded and discuss with a colleague how they might have been avoided. Is there any particular trend, eg falls or injury due to a particular treatment?

First aid

Someone in the salon should be trained in First Aid. Your local St Johns Ambulance (St Andrews Ambulance in Scotland) or Red Cross will be able to give you details of courses.

The first aid box

The trained first aider will have responsibility for ensuring that the first aid box is adequately stocked. The first aid box should contain:

- assorted plasters individually wrapped
- triangular bandages
- sterile eye pads
- different sizes of sterile dressings
- safety pins.

NOTE! Pain killers should not be issued by a first aider and therefore should not be part of the first aid kit. Antiseptics should not be part of the first aid kit because, if they have been used previously and the top not secured, they may contain germs.

First aid for minor accidents

It may be necessary for you to deal with minor accidents before calling upon the trained first aider.

- **Dizziness:** sit the person down near an open window for fresh air. Loosen clothing around the neck. Placing the head between the knees will help to bring blood to the head but care must be taken with elderly people.
- **Fainting:** as above, but if possible lie the person down with their legs raised.
- **Minor cuts:** apply pressure with a clean cotton wool. Follow procedure for handling contaminated materials on page 22.

- **Epilepsy:** a person suffering from an epileptic fit may injure themselves by falling or hitting furniture during an attack. Do not try to restrain them but ensure that their airways are clear. When the attack is over, cover the person with a blanket and allow them to rest.
- **Minor burns:** hold the area under cold running water until the pain is gone.
- **Nose bleed:** bend the head slightly forward and squeeze the bridge of the nose until bleeding has stopped.
- **Electric shock:** do not touch the person but disconnect the appliance at the mains immediately. Lie the person down and check their breathing.
- **Cosmetics in the eyes:** apply cotton wool soaked in water. Allow the person to wipe their eyes. It may be necessary to use warm water in an eye bath to flush out the eyes.

Element 1.2

Support health, safety and security at work

SAFE WORKING CONDITIONS

Heating and ventilation

The minimum temperature in the work place, by law should be 16°C (60°F). However the temperature in the salon should be around 20–23°C (68–78°F) as clients will be removing clothing. It is essential that the client is warm to encourage relaxation. An exercise room would need to be maintained at a lower temperature, around 17°C (63°F).

Thermostatically controlled heating will ensure that the salon remains at a constant temperature. Make sure that you know how to control the heating.

Adequate ventilation is equally important. Extractor fans and open windows will help remove strong smells from cosmetic preparations, fumes from chemicals and remove stale air which is caused by a build up of carbon dioxide and pungent smells.

Exercise rooms and wet areas must have very efficient circulation of air and good extraction systems: air conditioning is ideal. Headaches, dizziness, nausea, fainting and fatigue can be the result of poor ventilation.

Lighting

All areas of the salon should be well lit, particularly stair ways and fire escapes. The treatment areas where cosmetics are to be used should have natural daylight to ensure that make-up colours are not distorted. Matching make-up with skin tones or the client's clothing is an important aspect of applying cosmetics. 'Daylight' lamps can substitute for poor natural light where necessary.

Lights should be checked regularly, replacing flickering fluorescent tubes or changing the angle of lights which cause unnecessary glare.

Washing and toilet facilities

The law makes it very clear that an adequate supply of clean hot and cold water should be available in the work place, with separate washing facilities away from areas where food may be prepared or consumed.

The number of toilets is governed by the number of employees. A toilet must be available for clients. It is essential that toilets are spotlessly clean and checked regularly to ensure that there is a good supply of toilet tissue, hand towels and soap.

Salon cleaning

It is very important for the salon image, and to prevent the spread of infection, that the premises are kept very clean. Floors and windows should be cleaned once a week. This may be done by a cleaner employed out of business hours. Other daily cleaning jobs must form part of the salon routine, with all staff taking responsibility for completing jobs. This is usually done on a rota basis.

The Local Government (Miscellaneous Provisions) Act provides the Local Authority with powers to inspect the premises for hygiene and cleaning practices, in particular disposal of waste, cleanliness of floors, work surfaces and sterilising procedures.

Activity

1 It is essential that hygiene and safety tasks are carried out daily. Using the information contained in this unit devise a salon rota to ensure that all daily tasks are completed.

2 Use your rota to allocate tasks to the staff (students) in the salon and check at the end of the day that the jobs have been completed to your satisfaction.

3 You will need to discuss the rota with the manager and the staff. Outline how the jobs should be carried out and how you intend to check at the end of the day.

4 Remember to give feedback on how well the duties have been carried out.

> **Portfolio evidence**
> The rota is valuable evidence for your portfolio. Remember to get your lecturer or assessor to date and sign the rota, to observe you allocating jobs and monitoring that they have been carried out.

SALON DUTIES

General cleaning

Floors may be cleaned out of business hours, however it is important that any spillages are wiped up immediately. Wet floors should have a clear sign to stop people walking over them until the surface is dry and safe to walk on. Carpets should be vacuumed as required and any worn or frayed areas secured to avoid tripping.

Laundry

There must be sufficient clean towels, sheets and headbands to supply the salon. Laundry needs to be sorted and put into machines for washing regularly throughout the day. Washed towels need to be dried, folded neatly and stacked on shelves for easy access by the therapists. There should be sufficient washing powder and fabric softener available at all times. In order for the laundry to run efficiently, the machines must be in full working order.

> **NOTE!** Remember to note any electrical faults, switch off the machine, place a clear 'out of order' sign on the machine and report the defect to the salon manager immediately.

The salon may choose to send towels out to a commercial laundry. This will require counting soiled towels to go out and clean towels when they return. Paper work will need to be kept up to date to check the accuracy of invoices before payment.

Waste disposal

Each work area must have a small waste bin with a lid and a foot pedal for easy opening. Used cotton wool and tissues must be placed in the bin, not left lying on the trolley, couch or floor. This bin should be emptied after each client into a large receptacle for disposal at the end of every day.

Specialist waste such as disposable epilation probes are placed in a special yellow plastic container called a **sharps box**. This container must be handled with care and removed for incineration at appropriate intervals. Contaminated waste, i.e. with blood or serum on it, should be placed in a yellow bin liner for incineration.

Broken glass must be disposed of carefully by wrapping in newspaper before placing in the bin.

Basins and wet areas

Blocked basins must be dealt with immediately to avoid unpleasant smells. The 'S' bend under the basin has a screw cap which can be opened to remove blockages. Basins and shower cubicles must be wiped down after use with disinfectant. A ceramic cleaning fluid should be used at the end of the day to remove oil and lime scale. These can accumulate leaving unsightly stains which can harbour germs. Disinfectant should be poured down the drains at the end of every day. Saunas and steam baths require regular, thorough cleaning using disinfectant. The warmth and moisture provide the perfect breeding ground for germs.

Trolleys and work surfaces

Surfaces which are dusty and have creams, oils, or wax spilt on them look unsightly, unprofessional and will harbour infection. Spillages must be wiped up immediately and all work surfaces kept clean throughout the day.

Detergent will remove oils and creams. Products like depilatory bees wax should be left to cool, before being picked off the surface. Wipe over with surgical spirit.

Hand mirrors are often neglected and left smeared with finger prints. There is nothing worse than handing a dirty mirror to the client.

Equipment

Electrical equipment must be wiped over before and after use with a damp cloth to remove dust and any products which may have accumulated during treatment.

At the end of the day a final check must be made to ensure that all electrical appliances and salon equipment is switched off and disconnected.

Client refreshment facilities

Clients are often offered drinks or snacks in the salon. Hygiene procedures must be very strict when preparing food and drinks. If hot and cold drinks are supplied to the clients, they must be prepared in an area which is suitable, away from treatments and chemicals. The client should consume refreshments in a suitable room or rest area away from the treatment rooms. Disposable containers must be used if there are not adequate facilities for preparing drinks and washing up.

STERILISATION AND DISINFECTION

You must be aware of the importance of carrying out strict hygiene procedures to protect yourself, other therapists and clients from infection. There are guidelines laid down by the Local Government Miscellaneous Provisions act (see page 7) and Beauty Therapy Codes of Practice which outline hygiene procedures, particularly important when the treatment involves skin piercing (see page 27).

You must be able to recognise the skin disease and disorders associated with the area of the body you are treating (see Unit 5) and carry out the meticulous hygiene procedures which are outlined in this unit.

Infection

Infection is caused by micro-organisms which invade the body and cause inflammation. These include:

■ bacteria
■ viruses
■ fungi.

Bacteria

Bacteria can be thought of as those which cause disease, known as **pathogenic** and those that do not, known as **non-pathogenic**. They are categorised by their shape. Bacterial infection can usually be treated with antibiotics.

Cocci (singular = coccus)

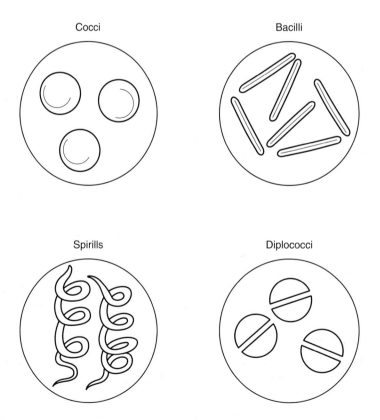

Figure 1.6 These types of bacteria can cause infection

Bacilli (singular = bacillus)

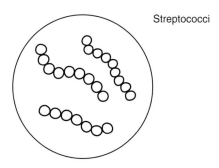

Streptococci

Spirilla (singular = spirillum)

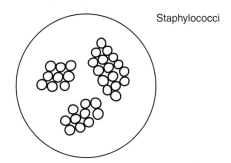

Staphylococci

Fungi

Fungi can be thought of as those which live on decaying or dead matter, known as **saprophytic** and those that live on living matter, known as **parasitic**. Both types cause disease within the human body. For example: Tinea Capitis or ringworm of the scalp, Athlete's Foot or ringworm of the feet and Onychomycosis or ringworm of the nail.

Viruses

Viruses are smaller than bacteria and infections caused by them are more difficult to control as they are unaffected by antibiotics. Viral diseases can be divided into two main groups:

1 Highly infectious diseases

These are transmitted by direct contact through droplets of moisture or mucus from the nose or mouth. Measles and the common cold are passed on in this way, for example.

2 Infectious diseases

Here the transmission is not obvious, but can be by direct or indirect contact. Viral infections of the skin fall into this group, such as warts or herpes simplex (cold sores).

There are two, serious viral diseases that a beauty therapist should be aware of. They are **Acquired Immune Deficiency Syndrome (AIDS)** and **Hepatitis B**.

AIDS

The virus known as the human immunodeficiency virus (**HIV**) affects the body's natural defence or immune system, leaving it susceptible to attack from other diseases some of which can be fatal. The virus is transmitted within body fluids such as blood. An HIV positive person can remain without any symptoms of AIDS for several years. In fact, in the early stages of infection the virus can be present but remain undetected when tested. It is imperative that strict hygiene precautions are followed during all beauty therapy treatments but especially when performing treatments that may involve contact with body fluids. Waxing and eyebrow tweezing, for example, can draw blood. As yet, there is no cure for HIV infection and AIDS.

Hepatitis B

This is a viral disease of the liver which is also transmitted within body fluids. The virus is more infectious than HIV. This is because the virus is more resistant and is able to live outside the body for a considerable time. The disease is very debilitating and can be fatal. The same strict hygiene precautions should be taken to avoid cross infection with the Hepatitis B virus as with HIV.

Infestations

This is a term used to describe the transmission of diseases caused by small parasitic animals. The most common infestation is by **headlice**. These infect the scalp and are common in small children. The condition is spread directly by contact or by the communal use of brushes or towels.

Another condition that the therapist may come across is **scabies** where very small mites burrow through and along in the epidermis to lay their eggs. The condition can appear red with the presence of swelling and fine lines indicating where the mites have burrowed.

Cross infection

Micro-organisms which cause disease are usually spread by coming into direct contact with the source. Sources include contaminated blood, body fluids, pus, sores or infected skin cells. Unclean tools, shared towels, dirty work surfaces and unwashed hands can be a source of infection in the salon.

Good hygiene procedures and the use of disposable materials will ensure that risk to yourself and others can be minimised. Cuts on your hands must always be covered by a waterproof dressing to avoid secondary infection which can occur at the site of a wound.

Methods of sterilisation and disinfection

The terms **sterilisation** and **disinfection** are sometimes confused.

- Sterilisation destroys all micro-organisms using chemicals or high temperature.
- Disinfection inhibits the growth of disease-causing organisms (except spores) using chemical agents.
- Antiseptic is a dilute disinfectant for use on the skin.

Sterilisation methods are very harsh, using high temperature such as boiling or strong chemicals. Sterilisation, therefore, is not suitable for many materials. The skin cannot be sterilised without using special chemicals which would not be suitable for use in the salon. Unless items which have been sterilised are vacuum packed, they can easily be contaminated by organisms which are carried in the air.

The therapist will generally use disinfectants or antiseptics which will inhibit the growth of bacteria.

Sterilisation methods:

- The **autoclave** uses high pressure steaming at a minimum temperature of 126°C. Autoclaves for salon use are small compact units which provide sterilisation for small metal implements. They are safe and easy to use providing the manufacturers instructions are closely followed.
- The **bead steriliser** uses dry heat at a temperature of between 200–300°C. These have limited use in the salon due to the small area available at the correct temperature for sterilisation. Because of the risk of burns when the implements are removed, they need to be used with care.
- **Ultra-violet light steriliser** uses ultra-violet rays from a quartz mercury vapour lamp. This method is very limited because of the need to turn the implements over to expose each surface to the rays. The cabinets do, however, provide a germ free environment to store previously sterilised implements.
- **Gamma radiation** is used for epilation needles at the point of manufacture. It is used under controlled conditions when large scale sterilisation is required.
- **Chemical agents** are available which, when diluted, can be used as sterilising fluids or disinfectants depending on the dilution. There are implications for health and safety in the salon due to the very toxic nature of the chemicals. A COSHH risk assessment would be required to ensure that special safety precautions are followed when preparing sterilising fluid for the salon (see page 5). Chemicals used are:
  - quaternary ammonium compound (QUATS)
  - gluteraldehyde
  - alcohol or surgical spirit.

> **NOTE!** Implements must be thoroughly cleaned by washing in hot soapy water before sterilisation.

Precautions to prevent the spread of infection

1. Cover any cuts or broken skin on the hands with a waterproof dressing.
2. Wear rubber gloves when carrying out any treatment where blood may be drawn to the surface of the skin.

Bleeding may occur during treatments where the skin is pierced or a needle is inserted into the hair follicle. For example:

- ear piercing
- epilation.

The therapist may also cause blood spots from the hair follicle during eyebrow shaping or depilatory waxing, particularly if very coarse hair is being removed such as with under arm or bikini line waxing. The coarse hairs grow from follicles which are deep within the dermis and surrounded by blood capillaries (see page 88). It is these capillaries which rupture as the hair is plucked from the follicle.

Dealing with blood spots requires very strict hygiene procedures to ensure that the therapist does not come into contact with the blood, to reduce the risk of infecting the client and to ensure that contaminated materials are disposed of correctly.

Procedure for dealing with blood spots or accidental cuts during treatment
1. Soak cotton wool in antiseptic or surgical spirit and apply pressure.
2. Place contaminated cotton wool in a contaminated waste bin inside a yellow bin liner.
3. Wash your hands.

> **NOTE!** The therapist may choose to take added precautions against infection by the Hepatitis B virus. It is possible to be vaccinated against this disease by a doctor.

HYGIENE CHECK LIST

Before the start of a treatment
1. Wipe the trolley with disinfectant and cover with disposable paper.
2. All tools which have been previously washed and sterilised must be placed on a clean tissue or in disinfectant on the trolley. Sponges can be placed in disinfectant such as 'Milton'.
3. Prepare the couch with clean laundry and disposable bed paper.
4. Check your appearance and wash hands thoroughly.
5. Carry out a close inspection of the client's skin in the area to be treated to check for contraindications.

During treatment
1. Ingredients are dispensed using a clean spatula onto the back of the hand or used from the spatula. This is known as a **cut-out technique**. (Fingers must not be dipped into products.)
2. All waste products must be placed immediately into a closed bin, preferably using a foot pedal to open it.
3. Apply all cosmetics with disposable applicators where possible.
4. If implements fall on the floor, wipe them over with disinfectant.
5. If you need to leave the client to do another job such as answer the phone, wash your hands before returning to the client.

On completion of the treatment

1. All implements are washed in hot soapy water to remove products and skin debris
2. The trolley is wiped over with disinfectant and prepared for the next client
3. Cosmetic jars and bottles are wiped and replaced in a closed cabinet
4. Sponges and brushes are washed in hot soapy water and rinsed in an antiseptic solution
5. All waste materials from the treatment area are disposed of in a lined covered bin
6. Soiled laundry is placed in a basket for laundering
7. The therapist washes her hands

SELF ASSESSMENT TEST

1. State four precautions which should be taken to avoid cross infection:
   a) before starting a treatment
   b) during a treatment
   c) after a treatment
2. What are the signs of infection?
3. What is the difference between sterilisation and disinfection?
4. What is cross infection?
5. Describe how facial sponges should be cared for to ensure that they do not harbour germs.
6. a) Why is the ultra-violet light method of sterilisation not satisfactory for sterilising salon implements?
   b) What use does the cabinet have in the salon?

PREPARING FOR TREATMENTS

Preparation before starting any treatment is essential to ensure that hygiene and safety procedures have been carried out. A treatment area must never show signs of the previous client: crumpled bed paper, used towels, used products left on the trolley.

Time must be allowed between treatments to:
1. prepare the treatment area
2. allow the therapist to check her appearance.

Preparing the treatment area

The appointment book will indicate what treatment(s) the client has requested. This may change after consultation with the client but the therapist can usually decide what clean laundry will be needed and how the couch, trolley and equipment can be set up.

Preparing the couch for facial and body treatment

A sheet and blanket with towels, a pillow and disposable bed paper will be needed. The clean items should be placed on the couch to form a 'cocoon' around the client which will be warm and provide adequate covering when clothing is removed.

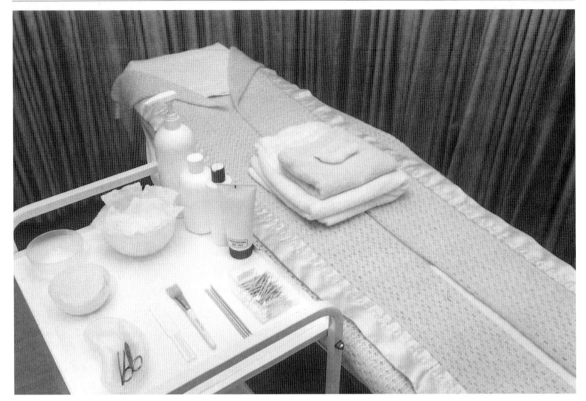

Figure 1.7 A couch prepared for a facial treatment

Preparing the trolley

Product trolleys, manicure trolleys and equipment trolleys must be wiped over with disinfectant and covered with disposable paper. Dust and spillages on trolleys can harbour infection and will give a very poor impression to the client. Bottle tops should be wiped, containers will need washing and a supply of dry and damp cotton wool and tissues will be required.

Preparing tools and equipment

Any item which is used on the client's skin has the potential to carry infection. Wherever possible such items should be disposable and thrown away after use, or be easily washed and sterilised or disinfected. Small tools and equipment such as tweezers should be wiped over or washed as appropriate and placed on the trolley in a jar containing disinfectant. Disposable items such as eye shadow applicators should be placed in the bin to be thrown away.

Facial sponges and cosmetic brushes can very easily harbour infection when they are left unwashed after use. The damp warm conditions encourage growth of micro-organisms. Sponges can smell sour if left dirty or placed in plastic bags. Whilst the use of sponges can be economical, saving on cotton wool, the chances of passing on infection is greatly increased.

Sponges and cosmetic brushes must be thoroughly washed in hot soapy water, rinsed in disinfectant solution, allowed to dry naturally and stored in an ultra-violet sterilisation unit or in an air tight container.

Personal presentation and hygiene

High standards of personal hygiene are essential to guard against cross infection and to protect the image of the salon. There are basic procedures which must be followed by the therapist:

- **Hair** must be clean, styled and away from the face. Constantly pushing the hair back during treatments is unhygienic and unprofessional.
- **Jewellery** should be kept to the minimum, particularly rings and bracelets which may come into contact with electrical equipment or the client.
- **Shoes** must be comfortable and appropriate for long hours of standing. Sloppy sandals or boots are not acceptable. Stockings or tights must be clean each day and free from unsightly snags or ladders. Keep a spare pair at work just in case.
- **Salon wear** will usually be a uniform and may be a full length overall or top, usually white or a pale shade, worn with trousers or skirts. Whatever choice of salon dress, it is important to have at least two overalls to allow for daily washing. Salon dress should not be worn outside the salon where it may pick up undesirable smells and become soiled.
- **Hands** must be well cared for, smooth with short manicured nails and no nail enamel. Dirt can become trapped under the nail and nail enamel can mask this, risking the spread of infection. Any cuts or sores on the hands must be covered with a surgical dressing to avoid cross-infection.
- **Fresh breath** is essential because of the close proximity to the client. Cigarettes and spicy foods containing garlic can taint the breath. They may be offensive to the client and should, therefore, be avoided. Brushing the teeth morning and night and after food removes particles of food and plaque which can cause bad breath. Bad breath (**halitosis**) may be the result of stomach disorders. Brushing the teeth or using a mouth wash whilst at work will help to avoid unpleasant mouth odour.
- **Body odour** (BO) is unacceptable and can be avoided by a daily shower or bath. Deodorants can help to maintain freshness, but remember they cannot cover up poor personal hygiene. Underwear must be changed daily and more often during the menstrual cycle when extra care must be taken to avoid unpleasant odour.
- **Day make-up** must be worn at all times when coming into contact with clients. It should be immaculate with particular attention to skin care. It is often the best way of selling cosmetics to a client. The client will expect to see the therapist practise what she preaches!

NOTE! The most important rule for the therapist is to avoid the spread of infection.

Thorough **washing of the hands** is essential before treating the client, after carrying out treatment and at any time during the day when the hands have come into contact with a possible source of infection, for example after visiting the toilet or carrying out cleaning tasks in the salon.

Washing the hands involves the use of hot water, soap or detergent, preferably antibacterial, thorough rubbing with the soap suds, followed by drying on a disposable towel. Special care must be taken to avoid contact with contaminated surfaces before starting work on the client.

Activity

Use the following check list to assess your appearance on a regular basis.

Personal hygiene and appearance check list

Is your salon uniform spotless and neatly ironed?

Is your hair clean and in a style which prevents your hair falling over your face during treatment?

Are you wearing comfortable, low-heeled shoes which are clean and not scuffed?

If you are wearing tights or stockings, are they changed every day and free from holes or ladders?

Are you wearing jewellery which may come into contact with equipment or the client, eg rings and bangles?

Have you brushed your teeth today?

Did you take a bath or shower before starting work today?

Are you wearing day make-up?

Does your make-up look professionally and carefully applied?

Did you wash your hands using hot soapy water and disposable towels to dry them, before and after treating your client?

> **NOTE!** You will come into close contact with your clients. Bad breath from smoking or spicy foods can be very offensive. Good personal hygiene is of the utmost importance to avoid unpleasant body odour.

Think ahead

The key to good preparation is to think ahead

- What do I need to carry out the treatment?
- Will my client be comfortable?
- Is the treatment area clean, tidy and hygienic?
- Have I accounted for likely hazards which may put me or my client at risk?
- Is my appearance immaculate and professional?

> **NOTE!** The preparation for specific treatments will be dealt with at the beginning of the relevant chapter.

SALON RULES AND REGULATIONS

Health and Safety legislation demands that employers set out **policies** on safe working practice. This will usually take the form of salon rules and regulations which are posted on notice boards in staff areas or as part of the employees' contract of employment.

Generally speaking the policies will follow the **codes of ethics** supplied by the various professional beauty therapy organisations as well as current legislation described in this chapter.

Rules will cover such things as:
- salon care and maintenance
- hygiene procedures
- fire precautions
- emergency procedures
- salon dress
- approach to clients
- safe working practices.

A code of ethics deals with the behaviour of the therapist towards clients, other beauty therapists and allied professionals through:
- referring clients as necessary to other professionals such as chiropodists
- upholding standards of treatment and not making false claims
- having loyalty to and respect for other beauty therapists by not criticising their work or 'poaching' their clients
- not gossiping or betraying the confidence of the clients.

A code of ethics will also ensure that the quality of treatment is maintained stipulating that:

- each client has a consultation to establish any contraindications and to find out requirements for treatment
- written permission is obtained from the client's doctor for certain treatments where the client's medication or condition requires it
- the therapist is competent and keeps up to date with the latest treatments
- the therapist does not make false claims and does not attempt to treat medical conditions.

A code of ethics will also ensure standards of health and safety are maintained by requiring that:

- practices and procedures are implemented and monitored
- staff are trained in safety procedures.

SALON SECURITY

Any business premises must have adequate security to ensure the safety of the employees and customers as well as to protect the property and contents. It is possible to insure against burglary and theft but the insurance company will demand that strict security procedures are in place to cover the premises both during business hours and when the salon is closed.

Security will cover:
- premises
- money
- stock
- personal property.

Premises

The salon owner should take steps to ensure that the premises are as secure as possible by:

- installing a burglar alarm
- fitting window locks
- ensuring door locks are of good quality and that bolts are installed
- fitting double glazing or toughened glass
- providing night lighting to give a clear view of the premises both inside and out.

Security procedures

1. Key holders should be kept to the minimum, preferably just the owner and/or the manager.
2. The police need to know who the key holders are in case of a break in.
3. A security check should be made at the end of every working day to ensure windows are locked, internal and external doors are locked, the alarm is switched on etc.
4. All staff must be vigilant of any breach in security, for example lost keys, broken locks.

Money

- Money should not be left on the premises overnight.
- The till drawer should be left open to show that it is empty.
- An electric till should be installed. This ensures that takings are locked away, that there are receipts and a record of transactions on the till roll.
- The salon owner will decide who has access to the till security code or keys and who is responsible for cashing up at the end of the day. Any discrepancies should be dealt with immediately.

Stock

- Stock must be kept in locked cupboards or a separate store room.
- A good stock control system gives a constant check on what is being used in the salon or sold to clients. Unfortunately petty pilfering can be a problem in the salon where staff may help themselves to stock. This can be kept to the minimum by a good stock control system.
- It may be that, on rare occasions, clients may take items of stock which are on display. This is regarded as shoplifting.
- Clients or staff caught stealing from the salon can be prosecuted and lose their job.

Personal property

It is not possible for the therapists or the salon owner to take responsibility for the personal possessions of clients. However as much care as possible should be taken to ensure that the client's clothing, jewellery and handbag are safe.

- Keeping possessions within sight of the client can be one solution, but it can be a nuisance to have things lying around the treatment area. An individual basket which fits under the couch for clothing and valuables is a good idea.
- Encourage your client not to wear lots of jewellery when she comes for treatment.
- Staff property should be placed in locked drawers or lockers may be provided. A changing area may be available if staff are expected to change in and out of salon uniform.
- Any security problems should be reported to the owner or manager immediately.
- Any insurance claim will require the police to be informed and full and accurate evidence provided.
- Visitors to the salon whether clients, tradesmen or casual callers can be potential security risks. They must be dealt with at reception and not allowed to wander around the salon unattended.
- All staff have a responsibility to care for their employer's property.

Giving evidence

If you witness a breach of security and the police are called, you may be required to give evidence. It is a good idea to complete an incident report form while the event is still fresh in your mind.

INCIDENT REPORT FORM

DATE	TIME	PLACE INCIDENT OCCURED

NAME OF INJURED PERSON	ADDRESS
	TEL. NO.

DESCRIPTION OF INCIDENT:

DETAILS OF ANY INJURY AND FIRST AID GIVEN:

SIGNATURE OF
INJURED PERSON . . . .

SIGNATURE OF PERSON
ATTENDING INCIDENT . . . .

Figure 1.8 An incident report form

Activity

Try to extend the following list of hazards in the salon by adding your own examples.

■ Slipping on wet floors or oil spilt on the floor

■ Tripping over trailing wires or loose carpet

■ Burns from hot wax

■ Scalds from hot water or steam

■ Allergic reaction to chemicals

■ Electric shock from exposed wiring or poorly maintained equipment

■ Cross infection from poor hygiene procedures or treating clients when infection is present

■ Drowsiness and fainting due to poor ventilation or fumes from toxic chemicals (eg nail extension products)

■ Fire from incorrect storage of flammable products or overloading of electrical circuits

■ Back strain from poor posture

Activity

1 Write down your responsibilities within the salon for security.

2 List what the salon rules are for care of clients' property.

3 Complete an incident report form (see page 30) for a real security incident you have witnessed in your salon. Alternatively, complete a form for an imaginary incident.

Portfolio evidence

Remember if you have carried out the procedures for a real incident get your teacher to date and sign the incident report form for your portfolio.

KEY SKILLS TASK

Allocating salon duties

The beauty therapy salon requires a team approach to ensure that the business runs smoothly, profitably and meets health and safety requirements.

The salon duties activity found on page 15 requires you to take responsibility for the allocation of salon duties to the staff team and to monitor performance.

Evidence produced by carrying out this activity will go towards assessment of key skills.

Working with others
Element 1 identify collective goals and responsibilities

Evidence Duties rota

Element 2 Work to collective goals

Evidence Feedback from colleagues on how well you worked with the team in allocating and monitoring salon duties

Information Technology
Elements 1, 2 and 3 Prepare, process and present information

Evidence Compiling a duties rota using appropriate software

Problem solving
Element 2 Select standard solutions to routine problems

Evidence Identify where the duties rota had to be changed due to staff absence or heavy work load, explain how you handled the situation and decided on an alternative strategy.

Communication
Element 1 Taking part in discussion

Evidence Discussions with the staff team to decide upon the needs of the salon and to ensure that tasks are completed

Element 2 Produce written materials

Evidence Produce a report to a senior member of staff to inform them about health and safety matters or on the way in which staff carry out salon roles for their appraisals

UNIT 2

Fulfil salon reception duties

In this unit you will learn about:

- the qualities of a receptionist
- interpersonal skills
- reception procedures
  - dealing with clients
  - answering the telephone
  - handling enquiries
  - giving information
  - taking messages
  - making appointments
  - dealing with payments.

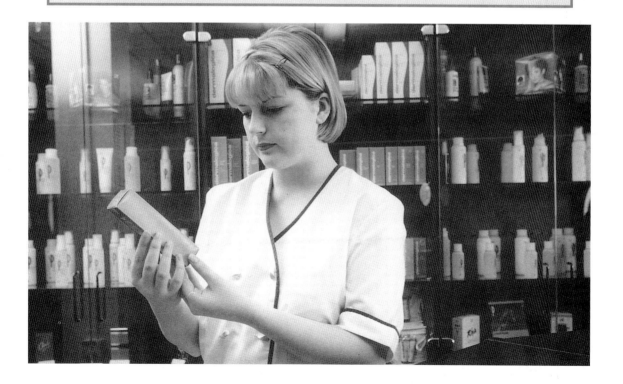

INTRODUCTION

Welcoming and receiving clients and visitors to the salon is an important part of the salon service. The client's **first impression** of the salon is given by the receptionist, whether on the telephone or in person.

All visitors and people making enquiries are potential clients. Therefore they must be treated in a **polite** and **helpful** manner.

Element 2.1
Attend to clients and enquiries

THE RECEPTIONIST

Qualities of a receptionist

Clients like to attend a beauty therapy salon to feel relaxed and to enjoy quality time in a pleasant environment. The receptionist can start the process the moment the client enters the salon by using her **interpersonal skills**:

- Make eye contact with the client.
- Smile and have a friendly manner.
- Be calm and gently spoken.
- Give the client individual attention and respect.
- Show genuine interest in the client.
- Be sensitive to the needs of clients and therapists.
- Take care not to do or say anything which could offend, particularly if it involves race, gender or religion.

The receptionist's role

Everyone working in a busy salon will have to carry out reception duties from time to time. So, it is important that all staff are aware of the procedures for dealing with clients and the manner in which they should be treated.

The reception area

This is the first part of the salon that the client comes into contact with. It must give a good

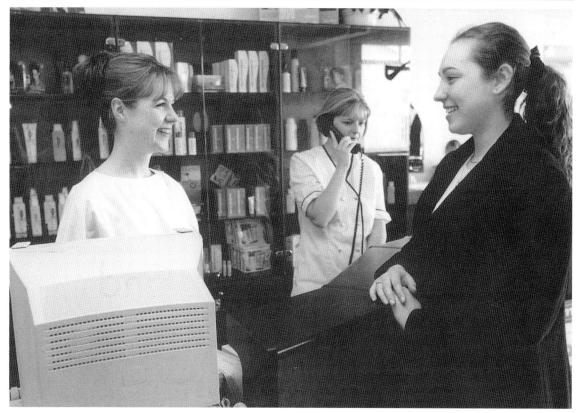

Figure 2.1 The reception area gives the client their first impression of the salon

impression by providing an area which reflects the high standards of hygiene and cleanliness, personal attention, comfort and relaxation which is associated with a beauty therapy salon.

The reception area must be kept clean and tidy by ensuring that:
- Carpets are vacuumed regularly.
- Retail displays are dusted and neatly arranged to attract the client's attention.
- There is a good supply of information leaflets.
- Used coffee cups etc. are removed.
- Flowers or plants are fresh and cared for.
- Magazines are kept up to date and stacked tidily.

Caring for the client
Welcome the client
The receptionist must make the client feel welcome by helping them with their coat and offering them a seat. Magazines should be available with an offer of coffee or other beverages. A drinks machine can be a very useful asset in a reception area allowing the client to help herself. This can save both the receptionist and the therapist time. Information on treatments should be readily available for the client to browse through.

Dealing with delays

Should there be any delay the client must be informed and given an estimate of how long the delay will be.

If there is any change to her appointment, she should be politely informed and offered alternatives.

Records

Clients records need to be available for the therapists. They should be updated and filed after use. Computer files also need updating as required.

Saying goodbye to the client

When the client is ready to leave, the receptionist must ensure that she has been offered another appointment and deal with any retail requirements. The clients should be helped with her coat and thanked as she leaves the salon.

Handling enquiries and giving information

Good **communication skills** are an essential part of the beauty therapist's job and the role of the receptionist.

Communication skills are used to give and receive information. They include:

- speaking clearly
- listening
- reading and writing
- use of body language
- personal presentation.

A potential client will usually require details of treatments and products available in the salon. The receptionist should be able to explain the benefits of a treatment, how long it will take and the cost. Treatment price lists or product leaflets can be offered to the client.

Information should be as accurate and as helpful as possible. It should be offered in a caring and discrete manner. If you do not know the answer to a question, ask another member of staff. Remember that some questions from a client enquiring about treatment may be of a sensitive nature and must therefore be handled carefully and referred to the most appropriate member of staff.

Confidentiality

Any information given by the client, perhaps for the record card or to do with the type of treatment she requests, must be treated as confidential. It should not be discussed, other than in a professional capacity, with other members of staff. Some treatments such as epilation (permanent hair removal) require detailed information on the client's health and medication. This information must be treated with sensitivity. Some clients requiring treatment for permanent hair removal may not wish other clients, who may be acquaintances, to know about it.

Some clients, wishing to be friendly, may involve you in gossip or 'tittle tattle'. Try to change the subject by choosing a more general topic. Never answer questions about other clients and always respond by saying that you do not have the information or that it would be inappropriate to answer the question. The best way to avoid difficult or unprofessional conversation is to remain business-like and deal only with the reception duties.

> **NOTE!** Being friendly does not require you to be familiar. Do not discuss your own personal details with the client.

Types of confidential information

- ■ client record cards
  - – name, address, telephone number
  - – medical information
  - – treatment information
- ■ client's financial transactions
  - – how much she spends
  - – how payment is made
- ■ information relating to the business
  - – salon financial matters
  - – treatment routines
  - – product formulations.

Such information must only be available to the business and its therapists. It should be kept in a locked filing cabinet. Computer records are strictly governed by the **Data Protection Act** (see page 71).

Answering the telephone

It is important to answer the telephone promptly on the second or third ring. The salon will usually have a standard response when answering the telephone. The name of the salon, your name and an offer of help should be included. You should answer with a friendly, clear and enthusiastic manner. A dull voice will give an impression of boredom and disinterest. Do not use slang and sloppy speech.

Listen carefully to what the client has to say and respond in a positive way either by making an appointment, answering a question, taking a message or by offering to call back if necessary. Repeat back to the caller the main points of the conversation such as their full name or initials (remember there are lots of Smiths), telephone number and the details of the appointment you have made for them. Always do something positive rather than say no or that you don't know. Use the client's name as you speak to her. Not only is this polite, but it will help you to remember her name in the future. Always end by thanking the client for calling.

> **NOTE!** Telephone manner is very important and requires practice to feel confident.

Answering machines

An answering machine is useful for the therapist who works alone and is unable to answer the telephone during treatments. It also allows clients to contact the salon out of hours to cancel appointments, make enquiries or request appointments. All messages should be dealt with promptly and those requiring a return call must be dealt with immediately.

Taking messages

It may not be possible for a client to speak to a particular member of staff, whether on the telephone or face to face. A receptionist must be able to take accurate information from the client and judge the urgency of the call. A message which is clearly an emergency must be dealt with immediately. All messages must be acted upon as soon as possible. Some messages may be confidential and will therefore require direct contact with the individual therapist concerned.

A system should be in place so that no message is overlooked. You might consider using a notice board in the staff room or behind the reception for messages, displayed so that they can be seen clearly. Message pads of bright coloured paper can be placed on the reception desk. Carbonised paper is useful as it ensures that there are two or more copies as a record of all messages received in the salon.

Activity

It is good practice to keep a record of all messages that you handle in case there is some problem. For example, if the message does not get to the intended person. Keep a copy of all messages taken at reception. Make sure you write the message clearly, date it and get your supervisor or assessor to authenticate by signing.

DEALING WITH PROBLEMS AND THE DISSATISFIED CLIENT

The receptionist has to handle a range of problems which can affect the smooth running of the salon, examples may include:

- a client who is late for her appointment
- a client who demands treatment that is not booked and therefore no time has been allowed
- a client who is dissatisfied with her treatment
- a therapist who is delayed taking her clients for treatment.

Each one of these situations needs to be handled sensitively. Listen to the client carefully without making judgements or excuses. In the case of a client who is late or where a treatment has been incorrectly booked, it will be necessary to speak to the therapist concerned to see if she has time to fit the client in to her appointments schedule. Do not attempt to make decisions without consulting the therapist.

If a client is complaining about a treatment, discuss the problem with the therapist concerned or senior member of staff straight away. Reassure the client that the matter will be dealt with. Do not try to make amends yourself by offering free treatment for example. This would be beyond the limits of your authority. The manager will follow the salon policy on complaints and decide what action should be taken.

Your job is to keep the client calm, ensuring that she is dealt with promptly. The complaint should be logged by recording the date, time, name of client, details of the problem, how it was handled and by whom.

It is sometimes necessary to provide support for the therapists when they are very busy and falling behind with their appointments. You may be required to:

- liaise with the therapist and client, keeping them both informed of any delay
- tidy or prepare work areas
- provide coffee and magazines for the client.

Element 2.2

Make appointments for salon services

BOOKING APPOINTMENTS

Perhaps the most complex and important job for the receptionist is booking appointments. Mistakes can cause frustration and delay to both therapists and clients and may lead to loss of takings. There is nothing more annoying for a client than to find that the appointment she booked has not been written down or that the information on her appointment card is incorrect. Equally, the therapist will not be pleased at the disruption this may cause to other clients during the day.

Each salon will have its own system of booking appointments but usually a special printed book or loose leaf sheets in a file are used. The appointment book is an important business record which must be retained for auditing purposes.

The receptionist must:

- ensure that there is a good supply of pencils, pens, appointment cards, an eraser, ruler, and message pads
- prepare appointment pages for several weeks in advance

- be aware of therapists' times in the salon, taking account of part-time staff, holidays and so on
- book all appointments in pencil so that they can be adjusted easily and neatly
- understand abbreviations and the timing of different treatments
- have a salon price list available
- be aware of individual clients and their special requirements
- know how to book courses of treatments and schedule follow up appointments
- work closely with the therapists, seeking their advice on how appointments and clients should be scheduled. Remember they will know the individual needs of their clients and how long they require to carry out treatments.

Abbreviations and timings used in booking appointments

Abbreviation	Meaning
DNA	did not attend
C	cancellation
✓	client arrived

Treatment	Abbreviation	Approximate Timing
Half leg wax using cool wax	1/2/Leg cool	30 mins
Under arm wax using hot wax	U/arm hot	15 mins
Manicure with paraffin wax treatment	Man/paraffin wax	45 mins
Cleanse with evening make up	Cleanse/eve m/up	1 hour
Eye lashes and brow tint	Lash/brow	30 mins
Full body massage	B/mass	1 hour
Eye brow shape	E/B	15 mins

8.30	Anna	June	Tmasyn	Julie			
a.m. **9.0**	Mrs Buckthorpe		Mrs Lawton				**9.0** a.m.
9.15	Facial	*Doctors*	Full leg	Mrs Marriot			9.15
9.30			Bikini	eb			9.30
9.45			u/arm	lash tint			9.45
10.0	Mrs Clay	Mrs Braithwaite		Yvonne			**10.0**
10.15	½ leg (532400)	Facial		½ leg *Hot*			10.15
10.30	e/b	0532 791897	Jayne Marshall	u/arm			10.30
10.45			(895870)	man			10.45
11.0	K Reynolds		Cleanse/m/up				**11.0**
11.15	cleanse/m/up		eb	Denise Sharpe			11.15
11.30	(895701)	Mrs Parkin		man/paraffin wax			11.30
11.45		man (544101)	Swift				11.45
12.0	Kristy	Ped	eb				**12.0**
12.15	Bridal m/up	½ leg	½ leg/u/arm				12.15
12.30	lash/brow		LUNCH	McKenna			12.30
12.45	man			Full leg (cool)			12.45
p.m. **1.0**				u/arm			**1.0** p.m.
1.15		Lunch					1.15
1.30				Sarah Gregson			1.30
1.45			Heidi	Facial			1.45
2.0	Lunch		Facial				**2.0**
2.15		Becca Raey					2.15
2.30		730295		Judi			2.30
2.45		Facial	Mrs Davies	½ leg (cool)			2.45
3.0	Mrs Baxter	Steam	Facial				**3.0**
3.15	Body Mass	½ leg					3.15
3.30				Dickinson			3.30
3.45		Mrs Harper		lash/brow			3.45
4.0	Parish	eb (355021)	Miss Holmes	(398366)			**4.0**
4.15	lash tint	lash tint	lash tint				4.15
4.30	leg wax \ B.trim		manicure				4.30
4.45							4.45
5.0		Briton	Joan				**5.0**
5.15		543624	consultation				5.15
5.30		½ leg/bikini					5.30
5.45		Ped					5.45
6.0							**6.0**
6.15							6.15
6.30							6.30
6.45							6.45
7.0							**7.0**

Late night   Date *24 August THURSDAY*

Figure 2.2 You must make neat entries into the appointments book

Activity

Student's log of activities whilst carrying out reception duties

LOG OF VISITORS TO RECEPTION Dates on reception	With appointments – name	Without appointments – name	Requiring salon services	Having business with the salon
New clients and visitors	1			
	2			
	3			
	4			
	5			
	6			
	7			
Existing clients and visitors	1			
	2			
	3			
	4			
	5			
	6			
	7			
	8			

Assessor/Supervisor Signature ....

Student Signature ....

Portfolio evidence

The reception log may go towards assessment evidence for your portfolio

Name of person requesting price lists	Name of person requiring information regarding services and products	Name of client booking a treatment	Communication with individuals on the premises

Complaints regarding services and products	Business calls from suppliers of goods and services	Person seeking employment, course details	Internal calls

Please note down the date and the person's name

Assessor/Supervisor Signature ....

Student Signature ....

Element 2.3

Handle payments from the clients for the purchase of services and retail products

OPERATING THE PAYMENT POINT

The duties carried out by the receptionist will ultimately affect the whole business. The care required when recording information whether it is client details on a record card, treatment information in the appointment book or accuracy in handling money is crucial to the business. The reception desk must be fully equipped to ensure time is not wasted searching for a pen for a client to write a cheque, for example.

The salon should have a policy and procedures for dealing with customers at the payment point. Advice on dealing with different payment methods is given on page 45.

EQUIPMENT AND MATERIALS

Stationery

A good supply of stationery is essential including ball point pens, pencils, spare till rolls, note pads, date stamp, salon name stamp.

> **NOTE!** A **calculator** is useful when using a manual till, for calculating VAT (Value Added Tax), or when totalling a number of retail items.

Cash float

A cash float in the till is necessary to ensure that there is sufficient change when dealing with cash transactions. The receptionist must make sure that there is change available throughout the day. This means thinking ahead and changing notes as necessary. Change may be kept in the business safe or you may have to make arrangements for change with a bank. It can be very annoying for the client to be kept waiting whilst the receptionist hunts for the correct change.

The cash float may also be used as **petty cash**. Petty cash is used for small incidental items such as fresh milk, postage stamps or cleaning materials. It is essential that receipts for petty cash purchases are retained for the salon accounts.

Credit card equipment

Credit card equipment is required if a salon chooses to accept credit cards. For a small salon, which only deals in small transactions, it may not be worth the fee which the credit card company requires. If the business is authorised to accept credit cards, vouchers and a transaction printer will be necessary.

The till
Computerised tills

Computerised systems which incorporate records of stock levels and clients for example may be used in large salons. The computer is usually attached to an automatic till which records the transaction, stores the money and produces the client receipt. Some salons may also have a facility on the till to take debit payment cards.

Electric tills

An automatic electric till is used by most salons. This records the transaction on a till roll as well as producing a receipt for the client. Cashing up is automatic on the press of a key and sub-totals can be made at any point in the day by pressing specific keys.

Manual tills

A manual till which is a lockable drawer may be all that is required in a small salon. The transaction must be recorded by hand. It is more likely that errors will occur with this system and there is more opportunity for pilfering.

> **NOTE!** Because of the different types of tills, payment methods and salon policy you will need to be trained in all aspects of payment procedures for your salon.

DEALING WITH PAYMENTS

The receptionist must be able to:
- handle a range of payment methods
  - personal cheques
  - credit cards
  - debit cards
  - cash
  - gift vouchers
- be accurate when totalling bills and giving change
- provide an itemised bill for the client
- issue receipts
- record the transaction.

Payments in cash

The basic procedure will be as follows:

- You will receive information from the therapist on the treatment the client has received. An itemised docket or bill is required. This may also include retail items. (Remember the retail payments will need to be recorded separately for auditing purposes.)
- Total the bill and inform the client of the cost.
- Key in the amount(s) into the till.
- If appropriate ask the client how she would like to pay.
- When payment is in cash accept the money and look carefully at the note(s) you have been given. There are special facilities for detecting forged notes. It is a good idea to place the note(s) on the till whilst you calculate the change.
- Count out the change into the client's hand and ask her to confirm that it is correct.
- Place the note(s) from the top of the till in the till drawer in the appropriate section and close it.
- Give the client a receipt and thank her.

Payments by cheque

The procedure is as follows:

- Before accepting a cheque make sure the client has a cheque guarantee card. This card guarantees payment up to a certain amount usually £50 or £100.
- Check the card details are valid (see diagram below).
- Write the card number on the back of the cheque.
- Make sure that the signature on the card matches the one on the cheque.

When receiving payment by cheque follow the details shown in the diagram below. Do not rush, take time to check all the details carefully. Remember a cheque which is made out incorrectly may result in the bank delaying payment or refusing to pay the money into the salon account.

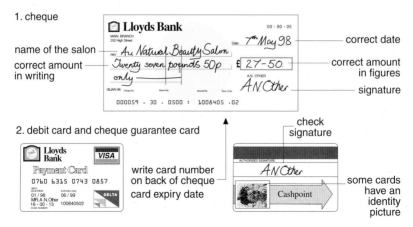

Figure 2.3 Check cheques and cheque guarantee cards carefully

Payments by credit card

To allow the salon to accept credit cards the salon must have an agreement with companies such as **Visa**, **Access** or **Mastercard**. A charge is made by the credit card company, usually a percentage of each transaction.

If a client wishes to pay by credit card the following procedure should be followed:
- Check the expiry date on the card. If it is out of date, do not accept it. Request some other form of payment.
- If the card is valid take a credit card voucher supplied by the credit card company (this is carbonised giving three copies). Using the card machine, imprint the card details onto the voucher. This will include the card number, which must be clearly visible.
- Complete the details of the service and the amount charged using a ball point pen.
- Ask the client to check the details and sign.
- Check the signature against the card. Return the card and the top copy of the voucher to the client.
- Place the copies in the till, one for the credit card company and one for the salon.

A computerised terminal may be used for credit cards and debit cards. The procedure to follow is described below.

Payments using debit cards

An electronic payment system such as **Switch** or **Connect** is used by many people instead of cash or cheque. The system uses debit cards which are issued by the bank. (These cards may also act as cheque guarantee card.)

You may be familiar with this system from supermarkets and other shops where payment points or checkouts have this facility. If the salon has a debit card terminal the procedure is as follows:
- The terminal is linked to a main computer which recognises the customer's card as it is 'swiped'.
- The details of the transaction are keyed into the terminal and a print out authorising payment direct from the customer's account is produced.
- The customer checks and signs the authorisation print out.
- The signature is checked against the card, a copy of the transaction and the card is returned to the customer.

Payment by gift voucher or discount voucher

Gift vouchers are **pre-paid vouchers** which are treated in the same way as cash. Most vouchers are dated to be used within a certain time, usually six months or a year from the date of purchase. The vouchers should indicate clearly the value and will usually be sold as £1, £5 or £10 'notes'. Each voucher should show the name of the salon, a signature and a number which corresponds with an entry in a book recording the date it was sold. This will guard against possible fraud.

Discount vouchers are a way of promoting salon services and may be part of an advertising campaign in the local paper: '£3 off when you spend £20 or more on presentation of this voucher' or 'a free manicure with every full facial on presentation of this voucher before Saturday 15th June'. These discount vouchers are a form of payment and must be collected for the salon records.

DEALING WITH INVALID PAYMENTS

In a busy environment such as the beauty therapy salon, mistakes can be made. These may not be noticed until the end of the day.

Discrepancies and invalid payments include:
- unsigned cheques
- incorrect date
- foreign currency (usually only small amounts in coins)
- out of date gift voucher
- incorrect adding up of a bill
- giving the wrong change
- pressing the wrong keys when entering amounts into the till.

These should be dealt with as soon as possible by contacting the client if appropriate. If an error, such as accepting a cheque without a cheque guarantee card has occurred, the cheque may 'bounce'. This happens if there are insufficient funds in the client's account and may lead to loss of the payment by the salon. The cheque can be presented to the bank again, but if there is no money in the client's account the salon must stand the loss.

Fortunately illegal transactions are not common but the receptionist must be aware of the possibility of a client using **forged** notes, a **stolen** credit card or cheque book.

If you have any doubt about the payment being made by a client, a senior member of staff should be called immediately. This must be done discreetly and without alarming the client.

The salon will usually have a **policy** on handling situations such as bad debts and fraudulent payments. Your job will be to take advice from the manager or senior therapist. Check what situations you have authority to deal with as they arise.

Activity

If, as part of your duties as a receptionist, you are required to 'cash up' at the end of the day keep a copy of the dockets or takings sheet.

Write a brief explanation of how your particular system of recording works. Remember there are many different methods of keeping financial records.

Get your supervisor or assessor to check the accuracy of your records and ask them to sign to show that all financial transactions that you were responsible for were correct for the day.

KEY SKILLS TASK

Reception duties

An important part of the beauty therapist's job is to handle the many tasks of the salon reception. It is usually only large organisations that have full-time receptionists.

Evidence produced by carrying out this activity will go towards the assessment of key skills.

1. Put together a weekly diary or log of all the jobs you undertake each day and keep together copies of information and materials which you use throughout the week. This could include messages, faxes, e-mails, samples of treatment dockets, cash sheets which you have added up and till receipts. It is important that you collect only materials which you have worked with and those should be authenticated by your supervisor on the day of the activity.

2. Keep a list of all the visitors to the reception (other than clients). Briefly describe how you handled different types of people, their business with the salon (example of a log can be found on page 43) and any problems you encountered. Include how you maintained security procedures with regards to visitors.

3. Keep a record of appointments you have made during the week using the salon appointment book. Clearly identify where you have handled cancellations, taken telephone appointments, informed staff about client delays or cancellations.

4. Maintain and update as necessary the client records file.

NOTE! Confidentiality must be maintained at all times. Do not divulge the business of your salon in your diary. Do not include detailed financial records and avoid writing full names of people you come into contact with.

Working with others

Elements 1 and 2 Work to collective goals and responsibilities

Evidence Keeping an appointment book, receiving visitors and keeping a register of visitors

Communication

Element 1 Taking part in discussion

Evidence Dealing with clients

Element 2 Produce written materials

Evidence Written messages, keeping client records

Element 4 Read and respond to written material

Evidence Receiving Faxes, e-males, written instructions

Application of number
Element 1 Collect and record data

Evidence Keeping records of takings throughout the day

Element 2 Tackle problems

Evidence Dealing with discrepancies, working out treatment cost

Problem solving
Element 1 Use established procedures to clarify routine problems

Evidence Extracts from the diary or log showing problems and how they were handled

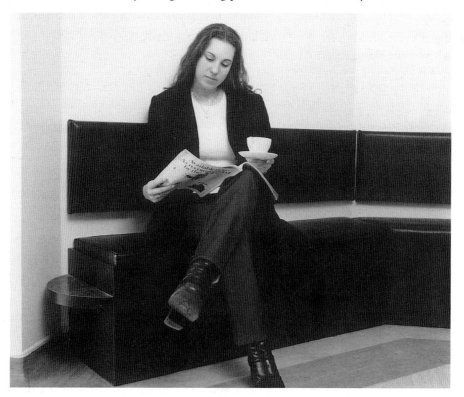

Figure 2.4 Always make the client feel comfortable

UNIT 3

Develop and maintain effective team work and relationships

In this unit you will learn about:

- working in a team
- the different roles and responsibilities of staff in the salon
- effective communication
- personal development
  - job description
  - appraisal
  - setting targets
  - reviewing personal progress and development.

INTRODUCTION

The success of any business depends on the way in which the staff work together to meet the aims of the business. Working as part of a team helps to spread the work load, promote good relationships with colleagues and ensure that the business runs smoothly.

Knowing what your role and responsibilities are within the salon is important to ensure that tasks are satisfactorily completed and that you can constantly review how effective you are and plan for your future development.

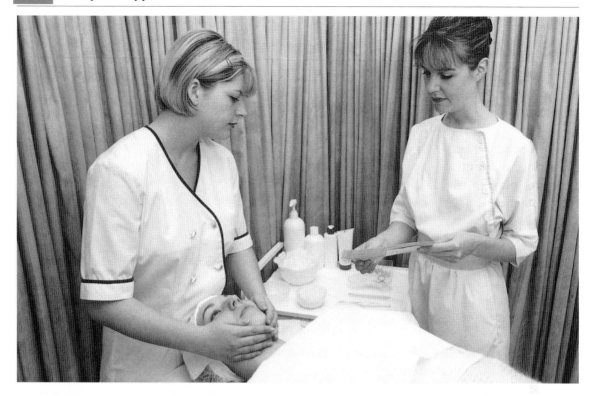

Element 3.1

Develop and maintain effective team work and relationships with colleagues

BEING PART OF A TEAM

You will at some time have experienced being in a team. This might have been in sport, hockey for example, in an orchestra or pop group, or as a member of the school play or local amateur dramatic society.

A team works to **agreed aims** or **goals**. A sports team aims to win a match, an orchestra or pop group aims to put together lots of different sounds from people playing many different instruments, a drama group aims to take different characters and put together a play or musical. This will involve a team of not only the actors but people to do makeup, costumes and lighting.

Many aspects of life involve working together as a team. This is particularly important in the work place. Whatever the business, be it manufacturing, retail or service industry it will rely on a team or teams of people working together to meet the aims of the company.

A beauty therapy salon is in the **service sector** of business with the broad aim of providing a range of beauty therapy treatments to its customers or clients. The salon owner will have a **business plan** in which the aims of the business are set out in more detail. The owner will require all the therapists to work together to achieve these aims.

BEING A TEAM MEMBER IN A BEAUTY SALON

You must be able to:
- anticipate the needs of others and be willing to **provide help and support** when it is needed
- **communicate effectively** and share information
- **get on** with all members of the team
- **accept responsibility** from your supervisor and work within the limits of your authority.

Providing help and support

When someone is very busy they can become flustered and agitated. As a good team member you will recognise that this person is under pressure and needs help. This may be something as simple as checking the temperature of the wax or preparing a treatment room for the next client. Anticipating when a job needs to be done and keeping an eye on those tasks which need to be carried out throughout the day are important aspects of your role.

> **NOTE!** Support staff in the salon are as important as the therapists themselves. The smooth running of the salon depends on their behind the scenes work.

Preparing treatment rooms or cubicles

Ensure that:
- equipment and materials from the previous client are cleared away
- the treatment couch is set up for the next client
- clean laundry is available
- products and equipment for the treatment are in place
- equipment is checked for safety and set up ready for the treatment
- the clients record card is available.

Care of clients and reception duties

The duties of the receptionist are described in more detail in Unit 2. However in a busy salon everyone must play a part to ensure that the client is cared for.

Unplanned situations such as late arrival of clients, overbooking of clients or staff absence will require you to use your initiative by providing the therapists with assistance and by ensuring that waiting clients are served with coffee, have a magazine to read and are kept informed. Clients who arrive without an appointment should be accommodated if at all possible. Remember this can give you the opportunity to provide the treatment yourself and gain a new client.

Housekeeping

Ensure that the salon is clean, tidy and running smoothly. This might include seeing to the laundry, doing some cleaning, sterilising and hygiene procedures, dispensary or stock room duties such as stock checks, dispensing or mixing treatment products.

Unit 1 deals with aspects of health and safety and salon care and maintenance. It also explains the importance of everyone taking responsibility for health and safety in the salon.

Communicating effectively

Communication is always important, not only between clients and staff, but also between staff and management and between the therapists themselves. Most beauty therapists are good communicators because of the demands of the job. They are able, through effective communication, to develop a good relationship with clients, provide professional advice and be a good listener.

Good communication between staff will ensure that everyone is clear about the aims of the business and their individual part in achieving those aims, as well as their role as part of the team.

Team meetings

Team meetings are a very good way of ensuring that there is effective communication. If held on a regular basis, they can help to:
- encourage and motivate staff
- provide training opportunities
- allocate tasks in the salon through negotiation
- identify and help to resolve problems
- avoid misunderstandings, disagreements or mistrust within the team
- provide an opportunity for the exchange of ideas for the future development of the business.

> **NOTE!** A good team leader (your supervisor or manager) will ensure that everyone is involved in the meetings, allowing open discussion of views and problems.

Methods of communicating in the salon

- ■ Written
  - messages
  - fax
  - e-mail
  - memorandum (memo)
  - appointment book
  - stock book
  - salon policies, rules and regulations
- ■ Verbal
  - team meetings
  - telephone
  - oral instructions
- ■ Visual
  - training videos
  - demonstrations
  - body language

Body language

Body language is a method of communicating. The wrong impression can be easily given by gestures, posture, facial expression and manner. A poor attitude will reflect in your appearance. Be aware of yourself and how you appear to others. A glum, stern face with the body posture in a slouching position with round shoulders will give totally the wrong impression. The therapist needs to be aware of her looks and posture. A bright smiling face which is well made up reflects the skin care and appearance of the beauty industry she wishes to promote. An alert body stance with good posture will give the impression of being ready to help the client and assist her with her appearance.

Activity

Put together a range of communication methods which you have used, for example a message, a fax, or an extract from the appointment book.

Remember for the evidence to be valid for assessment it must relate to an activity which you have carried out. It must be signed and dated by your assessor before you can use it as evidence for your portfolio.

Getting on with the team

Maintaining good relationships within the salon makes for a happy working environment. Clients can sense an atmosphere of discontent and disharmony, and this may put them off coming back. Building good relationships will require you to be aware of others; their needs, temperament, moods and to treat them with respect.

Accepting responsibility

Accepting responsibility for your actions and how you may affect others is an important aspect of life at work. It is essential to maintain the aims of the business, and to carry out your job effectively. An understanding of job roles and responsibilities within the business will help you to fit into the team by knowing what you are expected to do, who you should report to and who makes final decisions.

As an employee you should have a **job description** which outlines your work role and how you contribute to the overall work of the team. This needs to be reviewed as you gain experience.

Activity

There are many examples of team work. Working together in a group, discuss your involvement in a team and what responsibilities you had as part of that team. You might discuss your role in a previous job or in a sports team for example.

Element 3.2

Develop and improve personal effectiveness within the job role

THE JOB ROLE

The **job role** consists of the **duties** and **responsibilities** defined in the **job description**.

The job description

A job description will give details of your job, responsibilities and job title. A job description is necessary to enable you to define the limits of your authority: to ensure that you are aware of those things that are your responsibility but also where your responsibility ends. Further details of your job, such as hours of work, pay and holidays form part of your **contract of employment**.

Your job title will give you an indication of the level of your job (assistant, senior, manager).

Name: _____

Job title: _____

Place of work: _____

General description of the job:

_____
_____
_____
_____
_____

Responsible to:
■

Responsible for:
■
■
■
■

Main beauty therapy tasks (treatments):
■
■
■
■
■

Other tasks (general salon duties):
■
■
■
■
■

Figure 3.1 An example of a job description proforma

Salon Owner
Part-time therapist with regular clients
Works in the salon on Thursdays and Fridays
Only member of staff trained in advanced epilation, so has clients from the hospital
Responsible for: checking takings/till, banking, paying the wages, ordering stock, health
and safety, staff appraisals, staff training

↓

Manager/Senior Therapist
Full-time, six years' experience, works every day except Thursdays (unless the boss is
away)
Does all treatments and has a lot of regular clients
Responsible for: the day to day running of the salon and supervising the staff; client
records, appointment book, allocating salon duties, stock checks, health and safety checks,
staff rotas and holidays, daily cashing up
Responsible to: Salon Owner

↓

Beauty Therapist
Full-time, two years' experience
Building up her clientele, when not busy assists the Senior Therapist
Responsible for: daily hygiene practices and salon appearance, retail display, retail sales
figures
Responsible to: Senior Therapist and Owner

↓

Assistant Beauty Therapist
Part-time, recently qualified to NVQ Level 2, taking NVQ level 3 course part-time at
college
Manicurist and nail technician, waxing and make-up
Assists all the therapists by preparing treatment rooms, equipment and products
Responsible for: general cleaning duties including laundry, reception duties
Responsible to: Senior Therapist

↓

Trainee Beauty Therapist
Full-time, attends college 1 day per week for NVQ level 2
Assists all staff in the salon, observes treatments as appropriate
Responsible for: greeting clients, providing coffee, general cleaning duties
Responsible to: all therapists with training from the Senior Therapist

Figure 3.2 An example of a flow chart of staff roles and responsibilities

Activity

1 If you have already been in employment you will have had a job description and a contract of employment. Share your experience with someone in the group who may not have been in employment by discussing:
   - your job title
   - the job description
   - the tasks you were expected to carry out
   - who you were responsible to.
2 In your group use the proforma on page 57 to design a job description for a member of staff in a beauty therapy salon. To enable you to do this you will need to look at the staff in your salon or your work placement and make a flow chart of all the staff. Use the flow chart on page 58 to help you.

APPRAISAL AND PERSONAL DEVELOPMENT

Throughout your time at school, college or at work you will have been involved in **reviewing** and **checking** your performance and achievements. At school or college you may have experienced tutorials where you discuss your progress with your tutor and set targets for future learning, called an **action plan**. In employment, the tutorial is replaced by a **staff review** or **appraisal** which looks at your performance at work.

> **NOTE!** Whether you are having a tutorial or an appraisal, it is useful to think about the following questions:
> - **Where am I now?**
> - **Where do I want to be?**
> - **How am I going to get there?**

'Where do I want to be?' is when you ask yourself what your future aims are. Setting out your aims is important in all aspects of your life but particularly in relation to your career and future training needs.

'How am I going to get there?' is the point in an appraisal where you identify who can help you achieve your goals. During a staff appraisal the salon manager will discuss your strengths and weaknesses with you. You must be prepared to accept that they may have identified different strengths and weaknesses in relation to your performance in the salon. The manager may have different ideas for your future so it is important that an appraisal is a joint discussion with agreement on the goals and targets to be achieved. The question you need to ask is who and what will I need to help me to achieve my goals and targets. It is essential to put the goals and targets in writing so that they can be reviewed regularly.

'How am I doing?' is the question you should ask as you aim to achieve your goals and targets. After an agreed period of time your manager will review your targets with you.

Appraisal is sometimes referred to as a **review cycle** because each time the targets are reviewed and the goals and targets are achieved, the process starts again with new or modified goals and targets.

During the appraisal interview the appraiser who may be the manager or the person you are responsible to will encourage you to plan your training and development needs.

An **action plan** is agreed setting out your targets and what support you will need to achieve them. An action plan may include short-term targets, for example to practice using the new waxing system to be able to work on clients by next month, or long-term targets – to achieve the beauty therapy NVQ level 2 by July.

> **NOTE!** Appraisal is not just about identifying problems and planning how to solve them. It needs to be a positive process providing you and the manager with the opportunity to discuss all aspects of your job role. Targets which you set together should be written down on an action plan. They must be achievable and completed within an agreed time scale.

The date to review your targets will be agreed on the action plan and a copy retained by your appraiser. You will need to refer to the action plan to ensure that you stay on course to achieve your targets.

To enable you to plan for the future, whether in your career in beauty therapy or in your everyday life, you will need to set targets or goals. This will give you the encouragement and motivation to work hard to achieve these targets.

Managers in business use staff reviews or appraisals to evaluate the effectiveness of the whole work team. During an appraisal, you and your manager (in an interview situation) review your progress and contribution to the performance of the salon against the targets of the business and your personal goals. As well as thinking about your past performance, you will also look to the future. This will involve setting targets for your personal development, including training.

Appraisal

Self appraisal or appraisal with your manager will help you to manage yourself within your job role and to think about your future development.

You may find the questions listed above useful for appraisal. Begin with, 'Where am I now?'

To help you answer this question you will need to spend some time looking at your

strengths

- smart appearance
- good communication skills
- enjoy working with people

weaknesses

- not confident using electrical treatments
- need to be quicker with treatments

opportunities

- attending course at college for NVQ level 3 in September
- go to the trade shows in London

threats

- employed part time with little job security
- work in a small salon with only 2 other therapists who are also part time so do not get much time together

Figure 3.3 A SWOT Analysis

strengths and **weaknesses**. This is not always an easy thing to do as we are often more comfortable talking about our weaknesses rather than stressing our strengths. A useful exercise is to use the **SWOT** analysis. SWOT stands for **S**trengths, **W**eaknesses, **O**pportunities and **T**hreats.

Doing a SWOT analysis

1. Begin by making a list of the broad areas of your job such as assisting therapists with treatments and reception duties.
2. Then ask yourself, 'What do I do well and with confidence?' This will usually indicate your **strengths**.
3. Then ask yourself, 'What do I find difficult?' This will be things that you probably avoid doing or put off if you can. Things which make you feel anxious. This will be an indication of your **weaknesses**.
4. **Opportunities** will need to be considered through discussion with your manager during your appraisal. These refer to the limitations when setting targets. So, if you identify a weakness such as handling payments using the computerised system, this will require training. Therefore the opportunities for training will depend on the manager making the time available for you to go on a course or for someone to spend time with you in the salon for training.

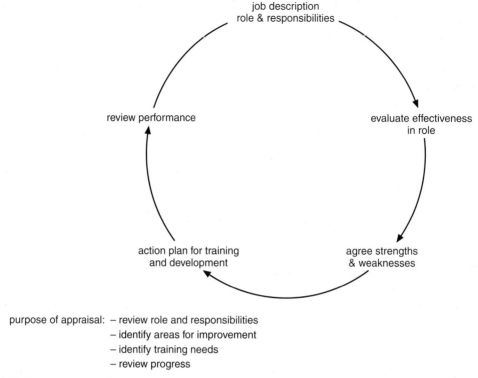

purpose of appraisal: – review role and responsibilities
– identify areas for improvement
– identify training needs
– review progress

Figure 3.4 An appraisal review cycle

5. The **threats** refer to the cost of such training and whether it would be cost effective to take time for this particular training need when there may be other priorities, training staff in the use of a new treatment for example.

The SWOT Analysis or any method of assessing your strengths and weaknesses will help you to monitor your progress and set your personal goals for the future.

TRAINING AND DEVELOPMENT

Beauty therapy is a fast-growing industry which requires the beauty therapist to be skilled in a wide range of treatments. The beauty therapist needs to keep up to date with new techniques, treatments and products, health and safety legislation and emerging technology.

Training needs of the staff will vary depending on their position, role and responsibilities within the salon. Training can include:

1. nationally recognised qualifications such as NVQs or equivalent vocational qualifications
2. manufacturers courses and information
3. keeping informed of the latest technology and trends through trade journals and professional bodies
4. in-house training to meet the needs of the salon, for example using a new product range

5. job shadowing allowing less experienced staff, possibly trainees, to observe treatments being carried out by senior therapists

6. management training for senior staff.

There is a constant flow of new products and techniques onto the market. It is important that you keep up to date with what is happening in beauty therapy to enable you to offer new treatments and retail new products to your clients.

Trade magazines and newsletters from professional bodies should be available in your salon as they are particularly useful for learning about the latest research and development in skin care, cosmetics and treatments. Trade fairs offer the very latest in products and equipment with demonstrations leaflets and free samples available.

KEY SKILLS TASK

Action planning and review

Planning for activities such as a holiday, a birthday party or a shopping trip requires some organisation and planning to ensure that everything runs smoothly. You will need to take account of what needs to happen (**target**) and by when (**time**). When the event is over you will look back on what happened (**review**) and perhaps decide to do some things differently.

On page 60 under appraisal a process of action planning is discussed in relation to your job role. You may begin by identifying your strengths and weaknesses. Using a similar process of planning prepare an action plan for your personal development over a two year period. This should relate to your future career.

If you have undergone an appraisal in your salon you may present the appraisal action plan as evidence for assessment in your key skills portfolio. You may also have a National Record of Achievement (NRA) from when you were at school. This will also contain evidence of planning for your future career.

Reviewing your action plan and amending your targets is an important part of the continuous cycle.

■ **Communication**

Element 1 Taking part in discussion

Evidence – Appraisal interview or tutorial

■ **Improving own learning and performance**

Element 1 Identify Targets

Evidence – Action plan for your future development

Element 2 Follow schedule to meet targets

Evidence – reviewing the action plan to see if targets are being met

UNIT 4

Develop and maintain positive working relationships with customers

In this unit you will learn about:

- service to clients
- approach to the client
- service standards and codes of practice
- professional practice and behaviour
- legislation relating to client treatment
- meeting client needs
- client feedback
- dealing with complaints
- client referral
- lines of communication
- client consultation and treatment planning

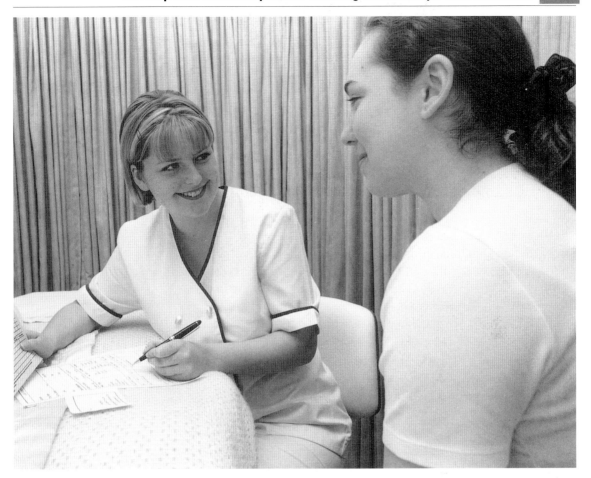

INTRODUCTION

The customer is at the centre of every beauty therapy business. Therefore it is necessary for the business to provide service of the highest quality to its customers, generally referred to as clients. The experience the client receives during her visit to the salon will influence whether she will return for further treatments and become a valued client.

Element 4.1

Present positive personal images to the customer

SERVICE TO THE CLIENT

The way in which the staff approach their jobs will influence the success of the business. Consideration should be given to the following:

- technical skills of the staff to provide efficient and effective treatments
- salon environment, decor and ambience
- professionalism of the staff
- health, safety and security in the salon.

The technical skills of the staff rely on good training through recognised qualifications and ongoing skills updating and experience. Treatments should be of the highest quality and should meet the client's needs as closely as possible. All work should be carried out efficiently and be cost effective.

The salon environment depends largely on the investment in the business by the salon owner(s) and the image they wish to project. Cleanliness is of utmost importance and this is reflected in the decor and care of fixtures, fittings and equipment of the salon.

The ambience of the salon will be very important to the client. Clients will wish to feel relaxed and comfortable in a peaceful and unhurried atmosphere.

The professionalism of the staff is important as it is they who contribute to the image of the salon and the quality of the treatments. Codes of practice provided by any one of the professional beauty therapy organisations give guidelines on the practice and procedures for treating the client. The salon will also set standards of appearance and behaviour for the therapists to follow which will take the form of salon rules and regulations. The therapist must aim to represent the salon in a positive way and follow standards of behaviour which comply with the organisation's service standards.

The responsibility for health, safety and security in the salon should be shared by all staff to ensure that clients are never put at risk. (See Unit 1.)

The following activity is designed to help you to consider how you would ensure that your client has a positive experience when she attends the salon.

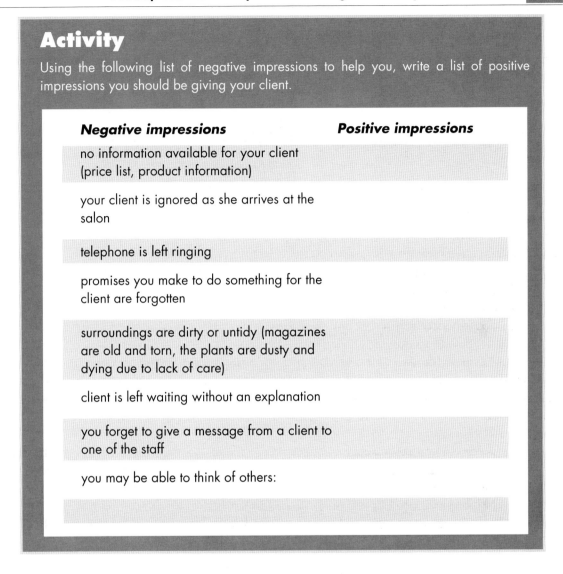

Activity

Using the following list of negative impressions to help you, write a list of positive impressions you should be giving your client.

Negative impressions	Positive impressions
no information available for your client (price list, product information)	
your client is ignored as she arrives at the salon	
telephone is left ringing	
promises you make to do something for the client are forgotten	
surroundings are dirty or untidy (magazines are old and torn, the plants are dusty and dying due to lack of care)	
client is left waiting without an explanation	
you forget to give a message from a client to one of the staff	
you may be able to think of others:	

SERVICE STANDARDS

Salon rules and regulations

The client's perceptions of you and the salon are very important. The image you project should follow the salon policy on standards of appearance and client care. The salon may have a manual or a notice in the staff room which outlines salon practice and procedures and rules and regulations. New members of staff will normally receive information on salon practice during their induction.

The professional way in which the salon staff approach their job will influence the success of the business. There are accepted standards of behaviour for the therapist outlined in the codes of practice supplied by the professional organisations. These guidelines may be adapted by a business to provide their own service standards.

The standards set by your salon or training organisation provide you with rules and regulations relating to:

1. Hygiene
2. Professional practice and behaviour
3. Dress
4. Treatments.

1 Hygiene

During your training you will be constantly reminded of the importance of hygiene and the need to carry out thorough hygiene procedures. The nature of beauty therapy requires close contact with the client and it carries the risk of cross infection. Clients have a right to expect high standards of hygiene throughout the treatment making cleanliness a priority for the salon.

There are new strains of viruses that are resistant to simple cleansing methods. This makes strict working practices a necessity (see Unit 1 for health and safety procedures).

- Cleaning equipment, **work surfaces** and **implements** should be part of your working routine. Ways of storing specialist equipment and safety checks are outlined in Unit 1.
- Fresh laundered **towels** and **bed linen** must be available at all times. Therefore, attending to laundry will be an important part of your salon duties.
- **Washing hands** is the simplest but one of the most effective hygiene procedures. It must become second nature to you to protect yourself from infection and also your clients and all those within the salon environment. Use **bactericidal hand wash** from a dispenser and water as hot as possible, followed by thorough drying with a disposable hand towel.
- **Cover cuts** or **abrasions** on your hands or the area to be treated on the client with a water proof plaster.
- **Wear rubber gloves** for treatments where there is any possibility of coming into contact with blood or body fluids (depilatory waxing, particularly under arm and bikini line waxing where blood spots during treatment are common). There is some concern about the possibility of passing on the HIV virus or Hepatitis through some treatments such as electrical epilation, ear piercing or where the skin can become broken. Studies have given contradicting information as to the risks, however procedures must minimise risk of cross infection from any source.
- **Sterilise** small implements using an autoclave or sterilising fluid.
- **Disposable items** such as paper towels, spatulas, tissues and cotton wool must be used where possible and disposed of immediately after use in a covered waste bin.

2 Professional practice and behaviour

The approach to the client is dealt with later in this unit, however acceptable standards of behaviour whilst in the working environment will include:

- speaking politely without the use of slang or bad language
- courtesy and regard for others
- no smoking, eating or chewing
- appropriate topics of conversation within the salon.

Behaviour is learnt from others and what may be acceptable for one person or within some work or social environments is not always appropriate for the beauty therapist.

Activity

Observe the way in which senior therapists who are experienced in working with clients in the salon behave. Use the headings on page 68 to check appropriate behaviour.

3 Dress

Salon dress or uniform should project an image of cleanliness and professionalism. White uniforms are the standard dress for beauty therapists with individual salons using coloured trim or badges as distinguishing features to promote the salon image. Smart shoes (not sandals due to the possibility of injury to the therapist's feet from equipment) with low heels should be worn.

Activity

Look through beauty therapy trade magazines or write to salon wear manufacturers for a brochure and select a uniform for your salon. Briefly describe the reasons for your choice.

4 Treatments

The therapist must keep up to date with professional practice and has a duty to find out about new treatments. Treatments are becoming more advanced with lasers and microcurrents being used to meet the demands of the client.

Professional qualifications, training courses, trade shows and trade magazines will keep the therapist up to date and ensure that treatments are performed to the highest possible standard. **Litigation** (legal action) resulting from alleged negligence by the therapist is becoming more common. It is therefore essential that the therapist is qualified and competent to practice.

PROFESSIONAL CODES OF PRACTICE

The **codes of practice** provided by the professional beauty therapy organisations lay down standards for their members including:

- **codes of ethics** – rules which aim to protect clients from improper practice. New members are usually required to sign an agreement that they will abide by the code of ethics.
- **professional codes of practice** which keep the therapist up to date with methods of treatment and procedures for beauty therapy such as hygiene practices new treatments and findings from research.

Failure to comply with your professional organisation's codes of ethics and practice can lead to expulsion from the organisation. Students of beauty therapy can apply for student membership and receive valuable information about events and new products and treatments.

Activity

1 What are the rules for your salon on dress and appearance? Refer to Unit 1 to check your appearance.

2 Ask to see the salon's service standards and make a check list for your staff notice board on salon rules and regulations. This should be well presented so that it is easy to read. Word process your check list if possible.

3 Contact one of the professional organisations and ask for information on their codes of practice.

LEGISLATION RELATING TO TREATING CLIENTS

Any person who buys goods or services is protected by the law to ensure that:

- goods are not faulty
- goods are of good quality
- there is an accurate description of the goods or service.

Legislation includes:

1. The Sale of Goods Act
2. The Supply of Goods Act
3. The Supply and Sale of Goods Act
4. The Consumer Protection Act
5. The Trades Description Act
6. The Data Protection Act.

1 The Sale of Goods Act 1979

This was the first of the laws which required **goods** to be accurately described without misleading the customer. The law takes into account the:

- suitability of the goods for a particular purpose
- quality
- description.

2 The Supply of Goods and Services Act 1982

This went further than the 1979 Act to include **standards of service** which should be:

- of reasonable quality
- described accurately
- fit for the intended purpose.

The Act also required that the service provided to a customer should be:
- carried out with reasonable skill and care
- within a reasonable time
- for a reasonable cost.

3 The Sale and Supply of Goods Act 1994

This amends the previous Acts by introducing guidelines on defining the **quality** of goods.

4 The Consumer Protection Act 1987

The European Community legislation provides consumers with protection when buying goods or services to ensure that products used on the client during treatment or retail products sold to the client are safe.

5 The Trades Description Act 1968, 1972

The Act protects the client from misleading descriptions or claims relating to treatments and retail products. For example, to claim that a treatment is a miracle cure which will prevent skin from ageing is not likely to be true and is therefore regarded as misleading.

6 The Data Protection Act 1984

The increase in the use of computers by businesses to store information about their clients has brought about a need for legislation to protect clients' personal information.

The Data Protection Act requires the business to be registered and to comply with rules on storage and security of data. Companies should:
- only hold information which is relevant
- allow individuals access to information held on them
- prevent unauthorised access to information.

The therapist and the law

The implications of the legislation for the therapist are clear. The customer or client has a right under the law to expect quality in respect of:
- the service they receive
- the products used during treatment
- the cosmetics or products that they purchase.

The therapist should be aware that not giving accurate information to the client or claiming that a product or treatment can do something which it clearly does not, is misleading and the client can demand her money back. If incorrect information is given, a product could be regarded as unfit for the purpose intended or not accurately described. The client must be reassured that information given during the consultation process is confidential and secure.

Element 4.2
Balance needs of customer and organisation

MEETING CLIENTS NEEDS AND EXPECTATIONS

Gaining feedback

The salon manager will need to be constantly aware of the clientele of the salon and whether they are satisfied with the services being offered. It is good practice to carry out surveys from time to time using questionnaires or comments cards. Anonymous feedback may give a more accurate response as some people are reluctant to make negative comments face to face.

Ways in which clients' comments can be collected:
- A suggestions box will encourage people to make comments.
- Comments cards can be left in the waiting area of reception. These cards could be like the ones you find at your table in restaurants like McDonalds or Pizza Hut.
- The therapist should make a point of asking the client at the end of the appointment whether she enjoyed the treatment and was satisfied with the result.
- The manager may use observation on a daily basis to gain information by checking the efficiency of appointment schedules, health and safety practice, client care or client satisfaction.
- Staff can contribute by listening to their clients and informing senior staff or the manager of any dissatisfaction or by making suggestions for improvement.
- Surveys or questionnaires can help to maintain and improve salon services as well as provide staff with valuable feedback on how they are doing within the team.

The manager will want to know that clients are being dealt with efficiently and that staff are meeting the targets of the business. Some clients with a negative attitude may use the opportunity to complain and criticise rather than make helpful suggestions. However, if there is a common thread running through the comments, it may indicate a need for action.

The salon manager may also wish to gain client feedback before a staff appraisal.

> **NOTE!** During **training** it is important for you to gain feedback from the client on your own performance. You may be asked by your assessor to keep a diary or log to record the treatments you do and the views of your clients.

Following up client feedback

It is always necessary to balance the needs of the client with what is viable for the business. To achieve this balance feedback from both clients and staff is essential. However, it is no good requesting suggestions and comments unless the information gained is acted upon.

Urgent action will be required where matters of health and safety, security or client distress are encountered. Non-urgent matters may be used to develop an **improvement plan**.

Comments from clients which will require urgent attention may include:
- 'The carpet is worn on the steps and I nearly tripped.'
- 'The temperature control on the shower is broken causing very hot water to come through.'
- 'The towels used for my treatment did not smell fresh.'
- 'The therapist was rude and abrupt when I phoned.'
- 'I was given the wrong change again today.'
- 'There is still no cleanser available for my skin type.'

It can be seen that these are matters of health and safety and service and must therefore be dealt with immediately.

The client may make comments on things which are desirable but not matters of urgency:
- 'I have read about a new face cream, are you going to stock it?'
- I wish you stayed open until 8.00 pm on Friday instead of Thursday.'
- 'I prefer fresh coffee rather than instant.'

It is not always possible to act on every piece of client feedback. The salon manager will have to consider whether suggestions for improvement are sensible and whether the business can afford to implement them. There may be implications for:
- financial investment in the salon for new equipment, products or staff
- staff training
- refurbishment.

Activity

Design a short questionnaire which could be given to clients to gain information on how satisfied they are with their salon visits.

Use the following headings to help you:
First impressions of the salon and staff
Salon appearance/decor
Hospitality and comfort
Enjoyment of treatment(s)
Value for money.

If possible, use your questionnaire to collect some views. You will need to type or word process the questionnaire and plan how it is to be issued to the clients. Completed questionnaires will need to be collected and the results analysed. From the results you may be able to make recommendations for improvement to the service your salon offers.

NOTE! As many clients as possible should complete the questionnaire to ensure that sufficient information is collected.

Activity

You may have experience from previous employment of dealing with clients or customers. The following list identifies the tasks involved in dealing with customers. Tick those which you have experienced. Write a short paragraph for each stating how you were involved and what you did in each case.

- dealing with enquiries on the telephone
- dealing with mail
- sending and receiving faxes or e-mail
- receiving customers
- writing memos
- dealing with complaints
- covering for absent colleagues
- dealing with lost property
- care of clients property
- taking action in the event of an accident or emergency
- selling products
- dealing with sales representatives
- participating in fire evacuation/security alert

If you are able to produce evidence from a previous employer that you carried out any of these tasks on a regular basis, the evidence may go towards assessment for this unit.

Element 4.3

Respond to feelings expressed by the customer

APPROACH TO THE CLIENT

The way in which you approach the client is important. Client care is an essential part of the beauty therapist's role from the moment a client makes an enquiry to the end of the treatment. You will be required to:

- listen carefully
- observe the client
- make appropriate conversation with the client
- offer advice
- provide one to one attention throughout the treatment.

> **NOTE!** The relationship you make with your client will influence the quality of the treatment and the client's enjoyment and satisfaction.

It is important that the therapist is aware of the client's feelings and makes the effort to build good relationships by:

1. Practising good communication skills
2. Empathising
3. Caring
4. Taking responsibility
5. Showing courtesy and respect.

1 Practising good communication skills

- listen carefully to the client and others
- question appropriately and in a sensitive manner
- write clearly using memos reports, messages etc.
- use non-verbal body language and facial expression
- make appropriate conversation with the client.

2 Empathising

Put yourself in your client's place. Everything you do should be seen from the client's point of view. The client may sometimes feel confused or anxious about her visit to the salon. It could be the first time she has had a treatment and she will naturally feel apprehensive about what it will involve. She may feel embarrassed about having to remove clothing or be concerned about whether the treatment will be uncomfortable.

You must make every effort to explain fully what will be involved, and avoid any embarrassment to the client by ensuring privacy and adequate covering to maintain her modesty. The following activity will help you to think about your feelings in a range of situations.

Activity

How do you feel when:

- you make a phone call and are left on hold for a long time with no explanation?
- you are kept waiting with no explanation or apology?
- a shop assistant ignores you when you are trying to buy something?
- someone is serving you whilst they have a conversation with someone else?
- someone looks angry and speaks aggressively to you?
- you arrive for an appointment to find that it has been changed to another time?
- someone promises to do something for you but forgets?
- people are giggling in front of you as if they are laughing at you?
- you try to explain something but the person does not seem to be listening?

You may be able to think of other situations.

Have you ever felt uncomfortable or embarrassed?

Choose two situations and write down or discuss with a partner how the person should have behaved to make you feel more comfortable.

3 Caring

This is a genuine feeling of wanting to help others by:

- being able to recognise when someone needs assistance
- showing a willingness to help clients and others (remember the client will observe how the staff work together)
- showing genuine concern for the well-being of the client
- ensuring that the client is not put at risk
- recognising when clients have special needs and offer assistance.

4 Taking responsibility

You will need to:

- make decisions or solve problems which affect your client, quickly and within the limits of your authority

- refer your client to a doctor or another therapist as necessary, without delaying or inconveniencing her
- avoid passing on problems to others because you cannot be bothered to handle the situation
- take ownership of a problem and resolve it in the best way you can.

Showing courtesy and respect

Being polite and showing respect for others is essential in all aspects of life. You should:

- be aware of others
- show tolerance for differing views and behaviour (different cultures, religions and background will influence behaviour)
- not judge others or view them as inferior because they may appear to be different to you.
- recognise that being tolerant and having respect for others does not mean that you have to compromise your own standards and beliefs.

DEALING WITH A CLIENT AND RECOGNISING FEELINGS

We all have days when we feel irritable, upset, confused or anxious. This is part of human nature. What is important is that you can recognise these feelings in yourself and in others and learn how to handle them. **Facial expressions** and **body language** can give a good indication of a person's mood or attitude.

Facial expressions

Facial expressions can show:

- sadness
- anger
- thinking
- confusion
- disgust
- anxiety.

Body language

The way in which you respond to the client when you recognise expression of feelings can affect the whole experience for the client and may influence whether they return to the salon for treatment in the future. Equally, the way in which you handle your own feelings by overcoming such things as anger, frustration and unhappiness for example, by presenting a professional image will influence how successful you will be as a beauty therapist. You will be expected to display a calm and efficient manner at all times.

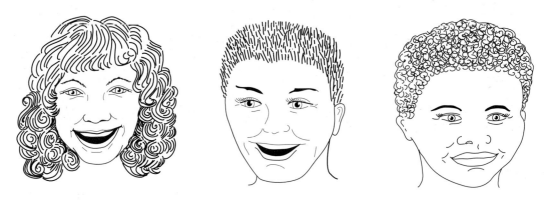

positive images
a bright smile, making eye contact, enjoyment in the job you are doing.

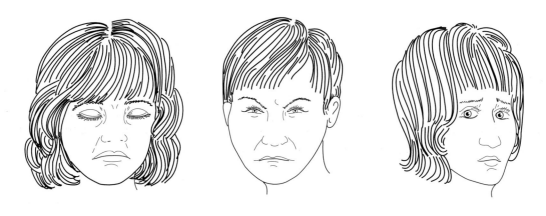

negative images
frowning, angry, avoiding eye contact, looking concerned.

Figure 4.1 Facial expressions give away a lot about your mood

Clients who are confused

It may be that the client has not visited the salon before or is having a new treatment. She may feel unsure and anxious about what to expect. You must recognise these feelings and give the client reassurance by explaining fully what the treatment involves, what she is expected to feel, making sure that she is comfortable and answering any questions she might have before you start. To enable you to reassure your client you must be confident in what you are doing and knowledgeable about the treatment. The manner in which you reassure your client should not be patronising, but aim to give her confidence in you and the salon.

Activity

Describe a situation when you have felt confused and unsure about what to do. This may have been your first day at college or when you have had to travel somewhere on your own for the first time.

■ How did it feel?

■ What would have made it easier for you to cope and feel more confident?

Challenging behaviour

The client may, in certain situations, display anger or aggression. This could be due to a range of reasons such as:

■ dissatisfaction with the treatment

■ poor communication where a situation has arisen because things were not clearly explained

■ the wrong attitude of a member of staff

■ the client may have personal problems which make her feel stressed.

Remember the client has a right to question what you are doing even though it can feel threatening for you. You must respond in a positive manner, without challenging the client or displaying anger. If at any time you feel that things are getting out of hand and beyond your control, excuse yourself and see a senior member of staff. This lapse in time can sometimes defuse the situation allowing space for the client to calm down and for you to regain your composure.

CLIENT COMPLAINTS

It is inevitable that there will be occasions when the client will make a complaint. These may include:

■ dissatisfaction with a salon treatment (a depilatory wax not completely removing leg hairs for example)

■ being kept waiting

■ an appointment mix-up.

A more serious complaint would involve damage to the clients clothing or injury to the client. Complaints may be made as they happen, verbally to the therapist or the client may request to see the manager. Alternatively clients may complain in writing after the incident. The salon may have a policy on the way in which a complaint should be handled. If so, this must be followed at all times.

NOTE! Any complaint must be taken seriously and rectified immediately.

A procedure for handling complaints

1. Listen attentively to what the client has to say, preferably in a private area. You may need to deal with the client's emotions first if she is angry or distressed. Acknowledge that she is upset and make her feel valued by showing genuine concern.

2. Decide whether it is within the limits of your authority to deal with the complaint following the salon's policy, or whether you should pass it on to a more senior member of staff.

3. A serious complaint carries a threat of litigation and must be referred to the manager who will make decisions on appropriate recompense or compensation. If the client wishes to take legal action there will need to be a formal record of events with witness statements and physical evidence of the complaint. Fortunately almost all complaints are fairly minor and can be handled by offering free treatment or by refunding the cost of the treatment.

    The client's rights are protected by the legislation relating to the consumer. Details of these Acts can be found on page 70.

CLIENT REFERRAL

It may be necessary to refer clients to other services within the salon or to recommend that they seek advice from other professionals, such as their GP or a chiropodist. A client may give details during the consultation of contraindications which prevent her from having treatment. You may need to advise the client to see her doctor.

For example, during a pedicure a client may ask you to remove hard skin on her toes. On examination you find the client has calluses and a corn which you are not qualified to treat. The salon may work closely with a chiropodist and refer the client by giving her a business card so that she can make contact herself.

A procedure for referral

The salon should have a policy on referral to ensure that staff are aware of the procedure:

1. A full consultation to check for contraindications must be given prior to every treatment.

2. The therapist must be able to recognise infectious skin conditions, skin diseases and other disorders and establish what constitutes a contraindication to treatment.

3. Clients should be directed clearly towards medical advice where necessary.

4. Referral must be handled in a manner which is sensitive and on no account must a diagnosis be made by the therapist.

5. A letter from the client's doctor giving permission for a specific salon treatment may be necessary. This must be attached to the client's record card.

Activity

Think about how you would handle the following situations.

Case study 1

A client arrives at the salon reception where several other clients are waiting. She very loudly announces her dissatisfaction with a recent leg wax treatment. She mentions the therapist by name and complains about her directly. She asks you to make a comment on how good you think she is as a beauty therapist.

Case study 2

During a consultation when you ask your client for information on her general health she begins to give details of recent major surgery and becomes very upset.

Element 4.4

Adapt methods of communication to the customer

LINES OF COMMUNICATION

Communication can be seen as an essential part of the therapist's role and is vital for the efficient running of the salon. So, the way in which you communicate with your clients, colleagues and manager will affect the atmosphere and efficiency of the salon.

It is important to follow the agreed methods and lines of communication within the salon. Look at the lines of communication chart in Unit 2 (page 58).

Many of the problems which arise in the work place are caused by poor or inappropriate communication. For example, interrupting therapists with trivial matters when they are treating clients is not good practice. Neither is holding on to an important piece of information which may require urgent attention.

Systems must be in place to allow effective communication between salon staff and may include:

- messages using a dry wipe board
- pigeon holes for paper messages and information
- staff meetings
- minutes or notes from meetings
- newsletters.

Making conversation with your client

One of the most daunting tasks when training to be a beauty therapist is meeting clients and knowing what to talk about. Clients can be any age but young therapists may find it difficult to relate to the older person.

Conversation with the client is an essential part of the service offered and is part of:

- making the client feel welcome
- gaining important information during the consultation
- receiving feedback during and after the treatment as to ensure that the client is comfortable and satisfied.

> **NOTE!** Some clients see the opportunity to unwind and talk about their problems as part of the treatment, whilst others prefer to be quiet without unnecessary talking. It is your job to assess the client's needs and provide conversation or peace and quiet as appropriate.

Starting a conversation

1. Find out your client's name from the appointments book or ask the receptionist. Find out what treatment the client is booked for.
2. Greet the client by using their title and surname. First names are too familiar for a first meeting and should only be used if the client specifically asks you to (or you know them personally).
3. If the client comes to you regularly, you should try to recall things from her previous visit to start the conversation. For example:
   'How did you get on with the night cream you bought last time?'
   'What dress did you decide to wear last Friday night?'
4. The client record card can provide you with information which may help you to start the conversation. For example:
   'I see you have been using the new product range Mrs James, how are you liking it?'
   'Has your allergy settled down, Mrs Andrews?'

The British are renowned for discussing the weather perhaps because it is one of the easiest ways of breaking the ice! It will invariably lead to other topics of conversation.

We so often ask the question, 'How are you?' without expecting a detailed reply. Most people just say 'I'm fine'. Changing the question slightly will make it seem like a more genuine enquiry. This can lead to conversation and provide valuable information for the consultation. Try: 'It's nice to see you looking so well, did you have a good holiday?' or 'I am sorry you had to cancel your appointment last week are you feeling better?'

You will need to have some background information or to remember things about your client to ask these sorts of questions. If you have not met the client before, you could use general topics from the newspaper or television. Remember that you must not discuss other clients or gossip. In Unit 2 communication skills in relation to client reception are discussed.

CLIENT CONSULTATION

Consultation requires the therapist to listen carefully and use questioning in a sensitive manner to illicit the important information required before the client's treatment. Information is recorded on a client record card or computer data base. Client consultation for individual treatments can be found at the beginning of each relevant chapter. Client consultation must be part of every treatment to check for contraindications and to establish the needs of the client before carrying out a treatment.

Confidentiality

It is important that you observe strict rules on confidentiality when dealing with clients. Your discussions with the client should be discreet and, when appropriate, take place in private. You must never repeat what your client has discussed with you in confidence. In some circumstances it may be necessary for you to seek advice, making it necessary to discuss client details with your supervisor. This would be acceptable in a professional context, but you would need to ensure that it was carried out in a professional manner to maintain client confidence.

Junior staff should be instructed on the importance of confidentiality and follow salon rules on approach to clients and appropriate topics of conversation.

Client records

Client records are personal to the individual and should be kept in a locked filing cabinet. If stored on computer, you will need to comply with the Data Protection Act (see page 71) to ensure that personal details remain confidential at all times.

Consultation, treatment planning and treatment records are essential. These are discussed in more detail starting on page 103.

KEY SKILLS TASK

Client survey

Collecting clients' comments can be an effective way of evaluating how successfully the business provides a service to its clients and to find out if the salon is meeting the needs of its clientele.

You can also use client comments to help you to establish how successful you are in your treatments. These should be collected in your log or diary as well as through evaluation sheets after you have completed a course of treatment.

On page 73 is an activity which can provide evidence for assessment of key skills

Information Technology

Element 1 Prepare information

Evidence Design a questionnaire to gain information from your clients on a range of treatment, client care and service. Issue the questionnaire to as many clients as possible

Element 2 Process information

Evidence Evaluate the responses

Element 3 Present information

Evidence Produce a table or graph of findings

Communication

Element 1 Take part in discussion

Evidence Issuing evaluation sheets or questionnaires to the clients with an appropriate explanation

Application of number

Element 1 Collect and record data

Evidence Data from the questionnaire

UNIT 5

Enhance facial appearance using make-up techniques

In this unit you will learn about:

- the skin
  - function
  - structure
  - disorders and diseases
  - damage
- preparing a treatment plan
- how to prepare for a make-up application
- how to select make-up products
- how to apply make-up.

INTRODUCTION

To obtain a perfect make-up finish, knowledge of the skin is essential. The beauty therapist must be able to make an accurate assessment of the client's skin in order to select the correct cleansing and make-up products, as well as the right application technique. Learning about skin disease and disorders is important, as the presence of a condition can determine whether a treatment should be performed.

> **NOTE!** Element 5.1 Assess clients and prepare treatment plans (page 103) applies to all units which deal with the technical skills needed to carry out treatments. These are Units 5, 6, 7, 8 and 9.

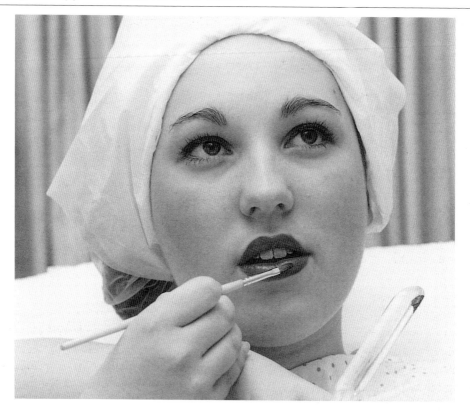

THE SKIN

The functions of the skin
Sensation
The skin is equipped with many sensory **nerve endings** making it sensitive to touch, differences in temperature, pain, itching, pressure and tickling.

Heat regulation
The body must maintain a temperature of 37°C in order to be healthy and the skin plays an important role in this. When we get too hot, the sweat glands in the skin produce sweat. This cools us down by using heat from the body to evaporate the sweat. The skin also becomes red (**erythema**). This is caused by the blood vessels near the surface of the skin **dilating** (widening) to allow more blood to come to the surface. As it does so, the heat is lost to the atmosphere. It is a little like a central heating system losing heat to a room through a radiator.

When the body is cold, the skin stops sweating and the blood vessels **constrict** (narrow) to keep the warmth in. Goose bumps occur as a result of each **arrector pili** muscle contracting and lifting its hair away from the skin to trap a layer of air. As we have very little hair on our bodies this doesn't work well in humans but is effective in animals such as cats.

The skin also stores excess food as fat which helps to keep us warm by insulating the body from the cold.

Absorption

The skin is able to absorb very little – its main function is as a protective barrier to keep things outside of the body. However, certain substances can pass through such as aromatherapy oils and small amounts of water. Cosmetic substances can be absorbed by the uppermost layers of the epidermis and sunlight can penetrate into the deeper layers if the skin is not properly protected.

Excretion

This is the removal of waste products from the body. The skin assists in this function by sweating through the pores in the skin which, as well as helping to control temperature, results in the removal of excess water and salts.

Secretion

Sebum is produced in special glands called **sebaceous glands** found in the deeper layers of the skin. It is an oil which flows out onto the skin surface, lubricating it and keeping it soft. When sebum is mixed with sweat it forms an 'acid mantle' making the skin waterproof. The face, chest and back have numerous sebaceous glands and can often appear shiny but soft and flexible. If excessive amounts of sebum are produced, the formation of blocked pores, **comedones** (blackheads) and **pustules** (spots) may occur.

Protection

The skin protects the body from injury and invasion by foreign bodies. The uppermost layers of the epidermis thicken with persistent pressure and are able to quickly replace themselves. The 'acid mantle' mentioned above is an invisible protective coat which makes the skin resistant to harmful bacteria.

The bottom most layer of the epidermis has specialised cells called **melanocytes** that produce **Melanin**, a pigment which darkens when exposed to ultra-violet light, protecting the dermis below it from the harmful effects of the sun.

Vitamin D production

Vitamin D is formed by the action of sunlight on the skin. It is then absorbed into the blood vessels and used by the body for the maintenance of the bones and the absorption of calcium and phosphorous in the diet.

The structure of the skin

The epidermis

This is the outermost layer of the skin nearest the surface. It is made up of five distinct layers and varies in thickness, being thinnest on the eyelids and lips and thickest on the soles of the feet and

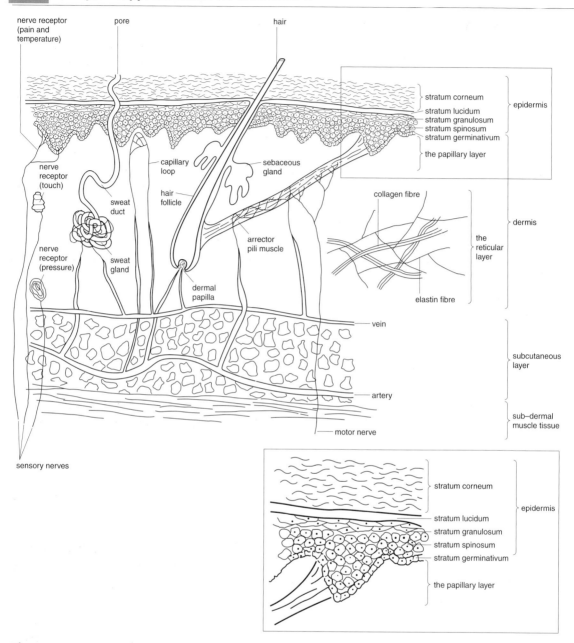

Figure 5.1 Structure of the skin

palms of the hands. The epidermis consists mainly of dead cells which are constantly being shed and replaced by new cells from underneath. The five layers are:

1. The **Stratum Germinativum** (the basal layer) – the cells are cube shaped, moist and obtain food and oxygen from the tissue fluid that seeps from the blood vessels in the **dermis**. This food and oxygen is used by the cells for division, a process called **mitosis**. As new cells are made, the old ones are pushed towards the surface.

   Special cells called **melanocytes** present in the stratum germinativum produce a pigment known as **melanin**. This gives the skin its colour and protects the underlying dermis from the harmful effects of ultra-violet light by absorbing the rays. Dark skins have many of these cells while fair skins have few. This explains why fair skinned people burn more easily in the sun.

2. The **Stratum Spinosum** – the cells here appear to grow spikes or spines hence the name. It is thought that at this point granules of melanin pass into cells from the melanocytes. The cells continue their journey towards the surface.

3. The **Stratum Granulosum** (the granular layer) – it is here that the cells begin a process called **keratinisation** which involves the formation of a protein called **keratin**. This causes the cells to harden and the nuclei to break down, leading to the drying out and death of the cells.

4. The **Stratum Lucidum** (the clear layer) – under a microscope this layer appears as a clear space within the epidermis. This is due to the absence of nuclei and cell walls. The melanin granules have been destroyed by enzymes and the cells are flat and filled with keratin, giving a semi-transparent appearance. This layer is thought to be responsible for controlling the passage of water in and out of the skin.

5. The **Stratum Corneum** (the horny layer) – the cells are now dead, flat, keratinised scales that are shed from the surface by natural rubbing from clothing and washing. When prolonged pressure is applied to the skin the stratum corneum thickens to form calluses which protect the underlying structures from harm.

It takes approximately one month from when a cell is formed in the stratum germinativum for it to reach the stratum corneum and be shed. This slows down with age, leading to the changed appearance of a mature skin.

The dermis

This layer lies beneath the epidermis and contains many different structures. It has the same thickness all over the body (approximately 3 mm) and can be divided into two areas.

1. The **Papillary Layer** – this is the uppermost area lying directly under the epidermis. Its name is derived from the projections that point upward into the epidermis called **papillae**. Some of these projections contain blood vessels providing food and oxygen to the germinating layer of the epidermis, while others contain nerve receptors giving the skin sensation.

2. The **Reticular Layer** – the lower area of the dermis contains a dense network of **collagen fibres** running parallel to the surface. Loosely woven between these are **elastic fibres**. Together these fibres give the skin its elasticity and if they are damaged by ultra-violet light, for example, premature ageing results.

    At the lowest part of the reticular layer is a network of connective tissue containing **fat cells**. This is known as the **subcutis** or **subcutaneous layer** which acts as a store of food and provides an insulating layer to keep us warm. This layer also provides some protection to the other tissues of the body by acting as a cushion.

The **dermis** contains glands and other structures that enable the skin to perform its functions. These structures include:

- **The Blood Supply** – A network of arteries run parallel to the skin's surface in the subcutaneous layer. Smaller vessels leave these at right angles upwards, towards the surface. Branches lead off to form capillary networks around **hair follicles**, sebaceous and sweat glands. These capillaries are responsible for taking vital food and oxygen to the living cells at the basal layer of the epidermis, the bulb and erector pilli muscle of the hair follicle and the sebaceous and sweat glands. Deoxygenated blood passes downwards through small vessels to the main venous network in the lower dermis. The amount of blood flowing to the surface of the skin is controlled by nerve endings in the artery walls.

- **The Lymph Capillaries** – there is a network of fine lymph vessels throughout the dermis which acts as a waste disposal system. The capillaries drain away tissue fluid containing waste products from cell activity and foreign bodies such as bacteria.

- **The Nerve Supply** – there are four sensations experienced through the skin. These are **touch**, **pressure**, **pain** and **temperature**. This is possible due to the network of **sensory nerves** and receptors in the skin. Most of the receptors lie deep in the dermis, but some that register pain can be found in the lower epidermis. All are stimulated by external influences, such as heat, and the message is taken along the sensory nerve to the central nervous system where the brain decides how to act upon the information. If it decides that action is necessary another message is sent along a **motor nerve** to an organ, gland or muscle. The message could cause the dilation of the blood vessels or the sweat glands to secrete sweat in order to cool the body temperature. It is along a motor nerve that a message travels causing the erector pilli muscle to contract to trap air next to the body for warmth and causing goose bumps.

- **The Sweat Glands** – there are two types of sweat gland in the skin. Both types are made up of a coiled body deep in the dermis and a long narrow tube or **duct** that passes up through the epidermis to the surface, where sweat is excreted through an opening called a **pore**. The **eccrine glands** are found in abundance all over the body and secrete water and salts. Their function is to regulate the body temperature. **Apocrine glands** are found in the armpits and genital area and open out into hair follicles instead of the skin's surface. They secrete water, salts, urea and fats. It is the breakdown of this type of sweat by bacteria that causes body odour.

- **The Hair Follicle** – this is a depression of epidermal cells pushed deep into the dermis. It is responsible for the production of a keratinised structure called **hair** from the **bulb** at the base of the follicle. The necessary food and oxygen required for hair growth is supplied by the blood vessels in the dermal papilla. Connected to the follicle is the erector pilli muscle which, when it contracts, pulls the follicle and therefore the hair into an upright position, causing goose bumps.

- **The Sebaceous Glands** – these glands are found all over the body, except the soles of the feet and palms of the hands. They are more numerous on the scalp, face, chest and back, with few being found at the knees and elbows. They commonly open out into a hair follicle but some open onto the skin surface. The glands produce an oil called **sebum** which lubricates the surface of the skin keeping it soft and supple and preventing moisture loss from the dermis. Together with sweat, sebum forms an invisible layer over the skin called the **acid mantle** which prevents attack from harmful bacteria and makes the skin waterproof. An increase in activity in the sebaceous glands results in a skin condition called **seborrhoea** or oily skin, which can lead to blocked pores, comedones and pustules. A decrease in gland activity will result in rough, dry skin and subsequent flaking and dehydration.

SKIN DISORDERS AND DISEASES

Some useful terms

- A **macule** is a small coloured area of skin that can be lighter or darker than the surrounding skin. It can be seen rather than felt. An **ephelides** (freckle) is an example.
- A **papule** is a small, solid, raised painful lump, red in colour and often develops into a pustule.
- A **pustule** develops from a papule and pus (which indicates infection is present) forms a yellow centre.
- A **vesicle** is a small, raised blister containing a watery substance called **serum**. It may be surrounded by an area of red skin and irritation.
- A **bulla** is a vesicle larger than 0.5 cm, commonly called a **blister**.
- A **nodule** is a small, rounded swelling either above or below the skin surface, also known as a **cyst**.
- A **tumour** is larger than a nodule and can be formed from hard or soft tissue.
- A **weal** appears as a white, raised area of indistinguishable shape surrounded by a red area. It may appear and disappear quickly, for example **hives**.
- **Scales** are used to describe flakes of easily detached skin, as with **psoriasis**.
- **Fissures** are cracks in the epidermis exposing the dermis.
- A **crust** results from the drying out of fluid from a lesion. Serum forms a yellow crust and blood forms a brown crust, called a **scab**.
- An **excoriation** results from the removal of the epidermis by friction also known as an **abrasion**.
- An **ulcer** is an extensive open sore with the resulting pus formation. It involves the epidermis and the dermis and healing results in scar formation.
- A **scar** is the replacement tissue formed during the healing of a wound.
- A **keloid** is an overgrown scar caused by the over development of collagen, common in black skins.

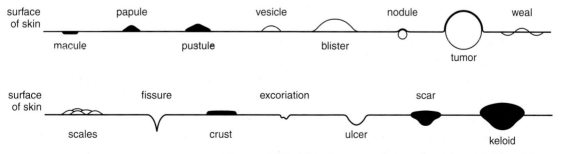

Figure 5.2 This diagram shows skin blemishes and lesions

Abnormalities of the sebaceous gland

Condition	Description	Appearance	Cause	Treatment
Seborrhoea	apparent in areas where sebaceous glands are prominent: the face, chest and back	excessive oilyness on the skin, pores become enlarged and blocked with sebum with the formation of blackheads – leads to acne	hormonal changes at puberty lead to over-active sebaceous glands	cleanse with the appropriate products, exfoliate and recommend the client have regular professional facials and use appropriate products at home
Comedones (blackheads)	associated with seborrhoea	small dark or black blockage in a pore	hardened, keratinised sebum blocks the hair follicle or pore, darkens due to the oxidation of the sebum in the air, can become inflamed leading to papules, pustules and acne	soften with steam and massage before extraction, advise client to cleanse with appropriate products, exfoliate and have regular professional facials
Milia	commonly found on fine skins in the cheek and eye area	white, pearl like nodules	sebum is trapped under the epidermis due to the pore or follicle opening being overgrown with stratum corneum	newly formed milia disperse with massage, if well established, can be removed with the help of a sterile probe or lance
Acne	there are various grades of acne some of which require medical attention – a doctor's approval must be sought before beginning treatment – commonly found in teenagers due to the hormone imbalance occurring at the time of puberty, but not limited to them alone, may affect the face, chest and back	excessive oil, comedones, papules pustules and scarring may be present depending on the severity	the pore or follicle becomes blocked with sebum and skin cells and yet the sebaceous gland continues to produce sebum which cannot escape anaerobic bacteria within the pore or follicle multiply and the structure becomes infected leading to the formation of pus the contents of the follicle may be pushed deeper into the dermis forming a cyst	if the client has sought medical attention, this will usually involve the use of antibiotics and the drugs Retin A or Accutane these drugs cause a variety of side effects such as dryness and sensitivity and so treatment by a therapist should be minimal at this time – after medical treatment the therapist can

Condition	Description	Appearance	Cause	Treatment
				treat the skin with caution as seborrheic and in consultation with the physician cystic acne should not be treated in the salon
Steatoma	commonly known as sebaceous cysts	soft or hard cyst varying in size from a pea to an egg	sebum is trapped within the gland due to a tightened or small opening into the follicle	steatoma are harmless and cosmetic treatments may be given unless there is infection present, medical attention is necessary for surgical removal
Rosacea	this condition seldom appears before the age of 30	inflammatory condition affecting the cheeks and nose, appears as temporary erythema and later flushing, becoming permanent, seborrhoea, papules and pustules are present in the area	unknown but is thought to relate to earlier seborrheic conditions in youth	medical referral is advisable, camouflage make-up can ease distress, advise client to avoid effectors of vasodilation such as spicy foods, heat and alcohol
Asteatosis	very dry skin which can be uncomfortable	flaky, dry skin with itching and cracking	under active sebaceous glands associated with the thyroid gland or old age	advise the use of emollient creams

Abnormalities of the sweat glands

Condition	Description	Appearance	Cause	Treatment
Hyperidrosis	excessive perspiration affecting the hands, feet and underarms where these glands are prolific		can be congenital but usually follows an emotional problem since the glands are controlled by the nervous system	frequent bathing, use of astringents and antiperspirant

| Prickly Heat | heat induced rash | small, red vesicles accompanied by itching and inflammation of the sweat glands | exposure to excessive heat such as the sun or sunbeds, sweat ducts get blocked by plugs of keratinised cells | frequent bathing in cool bath or shower, keep away from further heat, astringents can help |

Abnormalities associated with pigmentation

Condition	Description	Appearance	Cause	Treatment
Ephelides (freckles)	affect fair skinned people, found in abundance all over the body	small, brown macules which darken in sunlight and fade during the winter	congenital condition, inherited with the natural colouring	advise the use of a sunblock during exposure to sun, if disfiguring, can successfully be camouflaged with make-up
Lentigines	larger than a freckle	an area of brown pigmentation which does not darken in sunlight	congenital defect of the skin	camouflage make-up
Chloasma	common in women	light brown patches of pigmentation that darken with exposure to sunlight, vary in shape and size and can appear anywhere on the body but around the eyes, nipples and pubic area are common	melanocytes are stimulated by the increase in the hormone oestrogen during pregnancy and sometimes as a result of taking the contraceptive pill	the condition fades considerably after the birth or finishing the pill but a sunblock is advisable to avoid darkening, camouflage make-up is useful for facial cases, desquamation treatment can help.
Vitiligo	condition which is most obvious on dark skin	area of no pigmentation affecting the body or face and hair	the melanocytes are destroyed so no melanin is produced, can be congenital	use a sunblock on the affected areas, skin has a normal texture so camouflage make-up is successful

Pigmented Naevi	birthmark	large or small areas of light to dark brown pigmentation affecting any part of the body or face	congenital malformation	if on the face and causing distress camouflage make-up will help, raised naevi can be removed surgically if troublesome
Moles	very common type of blemish	vary in size, colour, and vascular appearance, can be raised or flat, found on the face or body, hair may grow from the affected area	congenital malformation	can be surgically removed if troublesome, if any changes occur to moles the client should be advised to see a physician
Albinism		pigment is absent throughout the body so an albino will have fair skin, white hair including the eyebrows and lashes and no colour to the eye	congenital defect where melanocytes are present but do not produce melanin	avoid sunlight and use a sunblock
Port Wine Stain	haemangioma disorders relate to vascular abnormalities	large, flat, red or purple area of permanently dilated capillaries, commonly found on the face	congenital defect that persists throughout life and does not fade	very effective results can be obtained with camouflage make-up and recently laser therapy has been developed that fades the blemish considerably, only available through a physician
Strawberry Mark	another vascular condition	bright red area seen at birth or shortly afterwards, soft to the touch and raised	multiplication of blood capillaries in the dermis	usually fades or disappears before adulthood, otherwise camouflage make-up is successful
Spider Naevi	vascular abnormality	a centrally dilated vessel with others radiating from it	associated with rise in oestrogen levels in pregnancy or liver disease	advise camouflage make-up techniques or diathermy coagulation by a trained electrologist

Abnormalities associated with skin growth

Condition	Description	Appearance	Cause	Treatment
Psoriasis	serious and irritating skin condition	oval or round shaped patches, raised and with the presence of silvery scales, patches have a distinct red outline and there may be some irritation if scratched, and the scales are removed then there will be bleeding commonly found on the knees, elbows, face and scalp but can appear anywhere on the body	faulty keratinisation of the skin cells and increased mitosis in the stratum germinativum, stress and anxiety worsen the condition	responds well to relaxation treatment such as massage and exposure to sunlight, medical attention is required in some cases depending on the severity, creams containing Vitamin A and/or steroids may be used. if no infection is present and the skin is unbroken normal cosmetic treatments can go ahead
Skin Tags	small growths	fibrous growth of skin tissue commonly found in the neck area, common in elderly clients and can be pigmented making them more obvious	excessive growth of the skin thought to be related to friction in the area	the attachment to the skin can be treated with diathermy under medical supervision but this does not prevent others from ar sing
Keloids	common on black skins	an overgrowth of scar tissue at the site of an injury	skin cells divide more fervently to compensate for the injured site	there is no treatment of this condition although surgery has been performed in severe cases and drugs administered to slow down skin growth, cosmetic treatments can go ahead as long as it does not aggravate the site of the blemish.

Other terms that are useful to know are:

- **Erythema** redness caused by the dilation of blood capillaries in the skin.
- **Hyperaemia** – an increase in blood flow to an area resulting in erythema.
- **Weeping** – a watery discharge from broken skin.
- **Oedema** – swelling of the tissue due to an accumulation of fluid.
- **Inflammation** – appears as red, painful swelling, warm to touch and followed by the formation of pus. Usually the result of bacterial invasion of the skin.
- **Bruising** – is an area of unbroken skin discoloured by blood from the damaged blood vessels in the dermis, usually as a result of a physical blow.

Skin blemishes and lesions

Blemishes may be present as a result of:

1. **Congenital malformation**, in other words, those existing at or from birth.
2. **Abnormal functioning** of the skin structures, those associated with the sebaceous glands, the sweat glands, pigmentation or with skin growth.
3. **Skin disease** by micro-organisms, bacteria, fungi or viruses.
4. **Damage** by external agents such as the sun, chemical trauma or physical trauma.

Congenital malformation

Malformations of structures within the skin at birth or shortly after will result in blemishes such as **birthmarks** which persist throughout life. These conditions can also be thought of as abnormalities.

Skin disease
Micro-organisms in the salon

Micro-organisms can be transmitted in the salon environment. They require warmth, moisture and food to multiply, all of which can be found in the salon. It is the therapist's duty to control the salon environment to prevent bacterial growth and cross infection. This involves hygiene and **sterilising procedures** and good **ventilation** through the salon. These measures ensure that the health of both the therapist and client is maintained. More details of suitable methods of sterilisation can be found in Unit 1.

Salon cleanliness

The micro-organisms which can cause disease are:

- Bacteria
- Fungi
- Viruses.

Infections caused by bacteria

Condition	Description	Appearance	Cause	Treatment
Folliculitis	small pus-filled spots	infection of a hair follicle with subsequent inflammation and pus formation	streptococci bacterial invasion of the follicle	the client should be referred to a physician, do not carry out any cosmetic treatments.
Furuncle	boil	acute pus formation involving the epidermis, dermis, subcutaneous tissue, hair follicles and sebaceous gland, with swelling, redness and pain as well as pus formation	staphylococci invasion through a cut or abrasion of the skin	requires medical attention probably the administration of antibiotics and lancing, do not perform cosmetic treatments in the affected area
Carbuncle	similar to a furuncle but more deep seated, requires medical attention			
Impetigo	highly contagious	vesicles which readily rupture to form a yellow crust	bacterial infection	medical attention is required, do not perform treatments
Conjunctivitis	highly contagious eye infection	the mucous membrane of the eye becomes inflamed and the eye appears red, puffy, weeping and feel gritty	bacterial infection of the membrane of the eye	medical attention is required, do not perform treatments
Stye		red swelling on the upper or lower eyelid at eyelash level, the eye may weep and pus is formed	the eyelash follicle becomes infected with streptococci bacteria	medical attention is required usually antibiotics and lancing.

Infections caused by fungi

All types of fungal infection of the skin and nails are types of ringworm (tinea). All types of ringworm are saprophytic (that is, they live on dead or decaying matter).

Condition	Description	Appearance	Cause	Treatment
Tinea Corporis	ringworm of the body	red, scaly, circular patches occurring on the trunk or limbs, spreading outwards, healing from the centre to give the ring appearance, vesicles and pustules can be present	common in pet owners as cats and dogs pick up the condition and easily transfer it to the arms and legs of their owners, highly contagious	medical attention is required involving the administration of a cream or tablets containing griseofulvin, do not perform treatments

The other types of ringworm that are commonly found are described fully in Unit 9.

Infection caused by viruses

Condition	Description	Appearance	Cause	Treatment
Herpes Simplex	cold sores	first sign is itching or burning of the skin around the mouth or nose area, followed by vesicle formation these weep or burst to form a crust which can easily split causing bleeding and scab formation, complete healing takes from 10–14 days	viral infection transmitted by contact either directly (eg kissing) or indirectly (eg drinking from the same glass) infection can reoccur as the virus lies dormant in the body until the body's resistance is low, some people say that the sun and wind can trigger an attack	medical attention can be sought for bad attacks but treatment is available over the counter in the form of anti-viral creams, do not perform treatments during an attack
Warts	highly contagious condition which can appear in different forms.	common warts – firm, raised, rough nodules of varying size, can have dark spots within the body of nodule flat warts – smooth, pearly elevations about pinhead in size. Found in groups on the hands and feet	viral infection passed on through contact	creams and lotions that contain salicylic acid can be bought over the counter, best removed under medical supervision, treatment can go ahead if the wart is covered with a waterproof dressing, if severe do not treat

SKIN DAMAGE

Damage by external agents
The sun

Condition	Description	Appearance	Cause	Treatment
Ageing	the sun can speed up the processes that occur naturally as skin ages	the skin appears leathery and will have many fine lines and wrinkles, elasticity is weak with the skin being slow to return to normal when stretched	ultra-violet light penetrates the epidermis and the dermis to the collagen and elastin fibres which are destroyed	exfoliate to remove the thickened epidermis and promote blood circulation, encourage growth of the collagen and elastin fibres with facials and suitable products, suggest specialist facials such as non-surgical facelift, galvanic and faradic treatments and encourage the client to use moisturisers and foundation containing sun protection factors at all times
Sunburn	skin can suffer long term damage following sunburn	the skin has an erythema with accompanying irritation and blistering, depending on the severity	ultra-violet light penetrates the epidermis to the level of the blood capillaries causing them to dilate, the longer the exposure the longer the capillaries remain dilated and so the erythema can last from several hours to days	soothe and cool the skin with cold water, rosewater or a mask made from calamine mixed with rosewater, if severe seek medical attention
Skin cancer	serious condition requiring medical attention	begins as a pale lesion, red patch or a mole that changes its appearance, for example getting larger, darker or becoming raised	it is not fully understood why cells become cancerous but it is known that the sun is the main cause of skin cancer, especially in areas of the world where there is a hole in the ozone layer	medical attention is required immediately, the client should seek a doctor's approval before any cosmetic treatment

Chemical trauma

Condition	Description	Appearance	Cause	Treatment
Dermatitis	allergic reaction to an irritant	red, dry, itchy area with the presence of papules and vesicles in severe cases, skin may crack and bleed leaving it open to infection by micro-organisms	prolonged contact with irritants such as detergents which break down the acid mantle, leaving the skin open to sensitivity	the condition is not contagious or infectious, so cosmetic treatment can go ahead if infection is present the client should seek medical attention and should also avoid contact with the irritant
Eczema	inherited allergic condition	similar to dermatitis in appearance but reoccurs throughout life	contact with an irritant can trigger an attack as can stress, thought to be a congenital condition, common in those who have a family history of hayfever or asthma	advise the client as for dermatitis, but in addition suggest stress-relieving massage if there is no infection present
Allergies	an allergic reaction can occur to many external and internal agents, the list includes cosmetics, washing powder and foods such as strawberries, heat and drugs	may begin as erythema, irritation or a burning feeling, if left untreated may develop into swelling or even blisters and weeping	which **allergen** triggers the reaction is dependent on the individual so it is important to ask the client if she has any known allergies it is possible that a client may develop an allergic reaction to an unknown substance during or after a treatment to avoid this, it is wise not to treat clients with several known allergens, in other words, one who is **hypersensitive** it is the therapist's duty to know the active ingredients of their treatment range	remove products from the area immediately with water only, continue to splash the area with cool water until symptoms subside. if they do not, the client should see a doctor as soon as possible

Physical trauma

Condition	Description	Appearance	Cause	Treatment
Broken Capillaries	common in fine and delicate skin types on the inner cheek and nose areas	fine, red lines in the skin surface	extremes in temperature, incorrect skincare, sunburn or physical pressure such as during extraction	protect the skin from the elements with moisturisers and foundation, treat gently during cosmetic treatment and camouflage using green corrective concealer, diathermy coagulation by a professional electrologist can be recommended
Urticaria	hives or nettle rash	red, itchy weal that can be localised or widespread, can appear and disappear within hours	allergic reaction to a foreign body causing the skin cells to release histamine, the allergen can be a food such as strawberries, an insect bite, pollen or drugs	the condition usually corrects itself within a few hours but may require medical attention if severe, do not perform treatments that may worsen the condition
Dark Circles under the eyes		darkness under or around the eyes	thought to be caused by a lack of sleep, but can be an inherited condition, can also be an indication of illness or oedema	a light covering of concealer can disguise the problem but the cause needs to be addressed if a cure is required.

Element 5.1

Assess clients and prepare treatment plans

INTRODUCTION

Each unit in this book which deals with the technical skills needed to carry out treatments refers to client consultation and treatment planning. This section of the book is about assessing the client and preparing a treatment plan. We aim to provide a general outline which can be applied to all clients for all treatments, not just facials.

At the start of every treatment, time must be allowed for client consultation. You should assess whether the treatment is suitable for the client and then prepare a plan of what the treatment involves. Sometimes a client will be offered a separate consultation to establish whether or not a particular condition can be treated in the salon.

To enable you to gain sufficient information during the consultation you will need to follow three stages:

1. **Questioning**.
2. **Visual check** – look closely at the area you will be treating and the overall appearance of your client.

contour brushes
these are used to apply
highlighter shades and
other corrective products.
The longest contour
brush is usually for powder
blusher application.

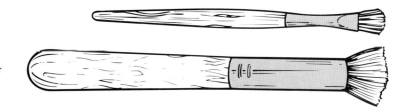

lip brush
this is used for applying
lip colour with accuracy.

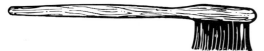

eyebrow brush
this is an essential brush
and should always be used.
Eyebrows should be brushed
as part of the general make-up
procedure to give a groomed
appearance. This brush should
also be used shaping the brows.

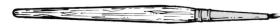

the **powder brush** is the
largest brush. It is used to
dust off excess powder following
application. By brushing upwards
and downwards, a velvety finish
is given to the skin.

an **eyeliner brush** is very
fine and can be used to apply
eyeliner with accuracy. It can
also be used for intricate
detailed corrective make-up.

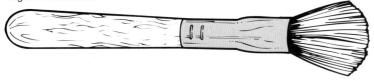

eyeshadow brushes
you should always have at least
two eyeshadow brushes. These
are used to apply and blend
eyeshadows. They are usually
square ended or tapered.

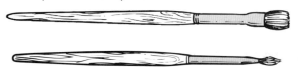

Figure 5.3 Different types of make-up brushes

3. **Manual examination** – touching the skin is important as it enables you to feel the texture and elasticity.

QUESTIONING THE CLIENT

Begin by explaining to the client what the treatment involves. This will help her to relax and gain confidence in you and what the treatment has to offer.

Questioning the client about requirements and expectations

Making sure that clients have realistic expectations of the treatment and the products is an important part of consultation. The client may have misinformed views on what can be achieved, or how she should be caring for herself. It may be that she has experienced pressure selling with over enthusiastic cosmetic sales assistants claiming that a product will do far more than is actually possible, or she may have read exaggerated articles in women's magazines. It is the job of the therapist to produce actual results by either improving the client's home care regime or changing her views on the benefits of good salon care.

> **NOTE!** It is against the law to make false claims (The Trades Description Act 1968 and 1972). Truthful and realistic outcomes are what matters if you are to keep your clients. Working together to change bad habits, to keep clients motivated and to keep them informed in best practice.

Where clients expectations are not achievable you should politely make alternative suggestions and give as much explanation as possible.

Question the client on home care routine

The way in which the client cares for herself between salon treatments is important information which is gathered during the consultation. It will give an indication of how committed the client is to skin care and health regimes, whether she spends time and money on herself and recognises the importance of visits to the beauty salon.

Question the client about her lifestyle

Selecting appropriate treatment for the client may be dependant on her needs at a particular time. This can be influenced by such things as her eating habits exercise and sleeping pattern, a busy life, whether she is happy and contented.

Question the client about previous salon treatments

These will be shown on the record card if the client visits your salon regularly. This is one of the reasons why record cards should be completed fully after every treatment and filed correctly for future reference. Any problems, such as adverse reactions to a treatment, can be recorded enabling you to establish appropriate treatment quickly and efficiently. If the client has had treatment at other salons it will be more difficult to gain information other than what the client tells you. You can, however, expect the client to be more relaxed if she has experienced salon treatments before.

Question the client about her general health

You should also ask about any medication she may be taking. Medical referral procedure should be followed when conditions are present which the therapist does not recognise as contraindications. The therapist must under no circumstances diagnose or make comment on any condition the client might present at the consultation.

Very often the relationship is such that the client may discuss a problem with the therapist rather than a member of her family. This is a difficult situation which must always be handled sensitively.

Examples of the sort of conditions you may come across relate to things like skin lesions, lumps or swelling or where a client is taking medication which causes skin irritation or rash. Under all such circumstances the client should contact her doctor and provide a letter advising you that it is safe to provide the treatment. This will also apply to long term health problems.

Most conditions, however, are temporary and you can advise the client to wait until the condition has cleared up before having treatment. On no account should the therapist make direct contact with the client's doctor by telephone or letter. The responsibility lies with the client, although you may wish to write down for her some details of the treatments or products you would be using.

Many conditions are localised: a verrucae on the foot would not prevent you from doing a manicure or facial on the client.

Discuss your recommendations for treatment

Use your skill and experience to ensure that the treatment relates to the individual needs of each client. The choice of product for treating the skin will depend on the client's skin type and the choice of depilatory wax method will depend on the client's hair growth. Explain your reasoning and provide an opportunity for the client to ask questions.

Use questions to clarify

It is important to ensure that details recorded on the record card are accurate and that the client is aware of what you have written. Give her the opportunity to read the details and to sign the card. This information is confidential and should be stored in a locked filing cabinet for access only by the beauty therapy staff. Information may be stored on a computer data base. This is governed by data protection laws.

Questioning techniques

- Ask appropriate questions which are not intrusive. It is not necessary to pry into your clients private affairs. It should only be necessary to ask general questions which allow the client to tell you as much or as little as she wants to.
- Ask questions in a tactful manner.
- Display empathy and understanding when questioning your client.
- Use open questions as much as possible to gain information.

Open and closed questions

With an open question, the client can give you a detailed answer. The answer to a closed question is either yes or no. Examples of open and closed questions which may be used in consultation are:

- Open question: 'Can you tell me about the skin care routine you follow at home?'
- Closed question: 'Do you cleanse your skin at home?'
- Open question: 'If you are taking any medication will you explain what condition it is for?'
- Closed question: 'Are you taking any medication?'

A VISUAL CHECK

The therapist should be prepared to look for signs of infection first and foremost, and then observe any abnormalities in the area. Whilst diagnosis of any condition is against the therapists' code of practice, you may need to make certain judgements about a skin lesion or unusual swelling, for example. The client will invariably be able to explain the condition and, providing you can establish that it is not a contraindication or that the treatment will not aggravate it in any way, you would be able to start the treatment.

Your assessment of the client will depend on a visual check of the condition of the area you are treating. This will enable you to select appropriate products and treatment. For example, you must establish the client's skin type before beginning a facial.

Observing the client as she arrives at the salon can help with your assessment, by giving you an indication of her temperament and attitude. If you are doing a make-up for the first time, it can be useful to look at the client's clothes, the colours she wears and how she does her own make-up.

You should observe your client's body language to see if she is relaxed or if she is uncomfortable.

FACIAL TREATMENT CARD

Name:

ADDRESS:

TEL: Work:
Home:

MEDICAL HISTORY:

MEDICATION:

DOB:

SKIN ASSESSMENT	date	date	date	date	date	date
SEBORRHOEA						
COMEDONES						
SENSITIVE						
MATURE						
SKIN COLOUR						
SUPERFLUOUS HAIR						
OTHER						
OPEN PORES						
ACNE						
DRY						
FLAKY						
DILATED CAPILLARIES						
SKIN BLEMISHES						
MILLIA						
SCARS						
DEHYDRATED						
LOSS OF FIRMNESS						
PIGMENTATION						
LINES/AGEING						

Client Signature   Date:

TREATMENT	Products used	Advised for Home Use	Products Purchased
Date			
1			
2			
3			
4			
5			
6			

Reassess the skin carefully after six treatments to judge changes in skin condition, success of home product use and make changes in salon and home routines as required.

Advised for   Products

TREATMENT		Products used	Home Use	Purchased
Date				
7				
8				
9				
10				
11				
12				

TREATMENT PROGRESS:

Client's comments:

HOME CARE CHECK LIST

Therapist Signature:

MANUAL EXAMINATION

Assess the client by touching the area to be treated to feel the skin's texture, or the warmth of the skin. When waxing establish the length and coarseness of the hair to be removed by touch.

It may be necessary to palpate the skin to feel muscle tone or to assess the elasticity of the skin. The therapist must be confident when touching the client and always have freshly washed hands.

MANNER AND ATTITUDE

A professional manner will require you to speak clearly, ask only appropriate questions, listen carefully to what the client has to say, and show respect. The way in which the consultation is carried out will give the client confidence and trust in your ability. Be prepared to give the client time to ask questions. It is important to build the relationship with your client and make her feel relaxed.

THE TREATMENT PLAN

The information gained throughout the consultation is used to establish the best course of action to meet the needs of the client. This is called a treatment plan.

Each treatment requires specific information and the detail appears in the relevant unit of this book. However, the general information which needs to be recorded includes:
- client's name, address and telephone number
- type of treatment and products
- area to be treated
- contraindications – notes on any medical referral
- any known contra-actions
- client's home care routine and any relevant information on lifestyle
- after care advice given and products purchased
- course of treatments – number and advanced payments
- outcome of treatment – results and effects
- client's comments and signature
- therapist's recommendations and signature.

The treatment plan should be ongoing and record progress over a period of time. Looking back over past records and seeing improvements can be very encouraging for the client.

INFORMING THE CLIENT OF COSTS AND TIME TAKEN FOR TREATMENT

The client will want to know how long she is expected to spend in the salon for treatment and how much it will cost. An up to date price list must be available in the salon. Should there be a change to the published prices, the client must be informed during the consultation. This will avoid any embarrassment when the client comes to pay. It is not good practice to spring extra cost on the client when you have completed the treatment.

The client should be given an estimated time for the treatment to be completed. This allows her to make arrangements and for you to keep to your appointments schedule. The therapist must be aware of time so that treatments are cost effective. For example, taking an hour to do a treatment which would usually be done in 45 minutes is not making the best use of time and your manager may question how efficient you are being. If, however, you are able to sell further treatments or products, this would be regarded favourably by your manager providing your next client is not kept waiting.

Courses of treatment paid for in advance offer financial benefits to the salon. A special offer for the client of one free treatment or a free skin care product can be an added incentive for her to attend the salon regularly.

SELLING

Beauty therapists must recognise that an important part of their role is to sell. This may be selling treatments, retail products or promotional packages for example. Therapists should be selling and promoting new treatments as they are introduced to the salon. They should also ensure that the client is aware that some salon services require a course of treatments. The application of individual false eyelashes will, for example, require the client to return for the lashes to be replaced periodically.

The client must be made aware of this during the initial consultation and it should be noted on the treatment plan. It is wise to offer courses of treatments as a whole package. This allows the salon to offer discounts and other incentives to the client. The client then understands exactly what it will cost both in monetary terms and in her time. You should also include any products required for home use in the total package.

HOME CARE

The client must be encouraged to undertake a home care routine. The importance of the home-care routine must be stressed if the treatment plan outcome is to be achieved. The client needs to be aware of what to do, what to use and when to use it. The use of a home care plan, which can be tailored to meet the individual requirements of the client, can assist in changing old routines and improving the skin condition. By including products which the client will need to purchase in with the cost of the course of treatments, a weekly cost could be given to the client which will include all her needs.

> **NOTE!** When selling treatments to the client always stress the positive end outcome: to achieve healthy strong nails, for example.

Activity

Make a list of the skills you will require to carry out a consultation and treatment plan, for example
- accuracy in writing down information

- empathy

SELF ASSESSMENT TEST

1. What is meant by medical referral?
2. What is meant by the term 'client's lifestyle'?
3. Give an example of each of the following when assessing the client for treatment:
   - an open question
   - a closed question.
4. List the general contraindications which prevent treatment.
5. Give two examples of contra-actions to treatment.
6. Why must client's details be recorded accurately on the record card?

Element 5.2

Prepare the work area and the client for the application of make-up

The use and effect of a professionally applied make-up should not be underestimated. Make-up is an important part of a facial but it is also becoming increasingly popular as a salon service in its own right. Many salons include make-up lessons as part of their menu of services. It is also a response to the growing demand for professional make-up application for weddings and portrait photography.

Make-up is used to 'say something' about the wearer. Therefore, it is vital to undertake a thorough consultation with the client to ascertain their needs and desires. A consultation also provides an opportunity to advise the client of achievable outcomes. All findings from the consultation should be recorded on the client's treatment plan (see page 103).

Make-up can be used, not only to improve and enhance, but to correct minor imperfections and to balance the features. Within most hospitals there are facilities available for cosmetic camouflage. Specialised make-up products and methods of application are used to effectively camouflage pigmentation abnormalities and skin disorders.

Specialised techniques are also used for photographic work, fashion and catwalk shows, stage, television and for creating special effects within television and film.

This unit, however, is dedicated to basic make-up product selection and application. Once these principles have been mastered, they will form the foundation for the further development of these skills. The art of make-up application is acquired through practice and experimentation with colour and different techniques.

PERSONAL PREPARATION

It is important to instil confidence in your client and as discussed in Unit 1 you must ensure your appearance is appropriate. A client will expect you to be professional both in appearance and manner. It is particularly important to wear make-up. This should not be heavy but will indicate that you take care with your appearance.

> **NOTE!** Remember to wash your hands before commencing treatments and to ensure that the client can see you doing this.

TOOLS AND EQUIPMENT

Lighting
One of the most important requirements for make-up application is good lighting. Ideally this should be **natural daylight**, however this is not always possible. You will need a good quality lamp, one that is capable of simulating natural daylight and that does not flood the face with bright white light. It should also be adjustable to accommodate client positioning.

Fluorescent lights should be avoided as should fixed lighting which may cast shadows on the face. It is important to ascertain the conditions in which the make-up will be worn and to adapt accordingly, for example you will have to consider the effects of artificial light on evening make-up.

Brushes
A good set of brushes will last for many years. You will soon find them familiar tools, ones that can be easily selected to meet the special need of particular make-up techniques. Professional brushes should be long handled and made from **sable** or **soft bristle**.

You will require a large-headed powder brush, a blusher brush, a contour brush and a selection of eyeshadow brushes. These should include a sponge-tipped applicator, an angled brush head, a dome-shaped brush head and a wider brush, which is useful for blending. You will find that most professional brushes will have the suggested function identified on the handle. You may disregard these if you wish and use whichever suits the need of the application. A combined brush/comb is required for grooming the brows and for separating the eyelashes. A fine brush is essential for eyeliner application and a lip brush is vital for applying cosmetics to the lips with precision. You will also require a selection of sponges and facial wedges. Eyelash curlers are another essential item as they enhance the eyes considerably.

> **NOTE!** Refer to Unit 1 for information on sterilising equipment.

You should also have a mirror available to show the client the finished make-up or to talk the client through each stage of a make-up lesson.

> **NOTE!** Remember to check for contraindications.

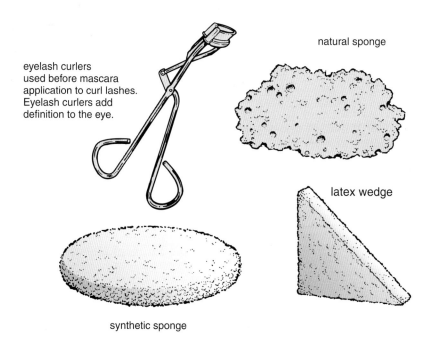

eyelash curlers used before mascara application to curl lashes. Eyelash curlers add definition to the eye.

natural sponge

latex wedge

synthetic sponge

Figure 5.4 Sponges, wedges and eyelash curlers

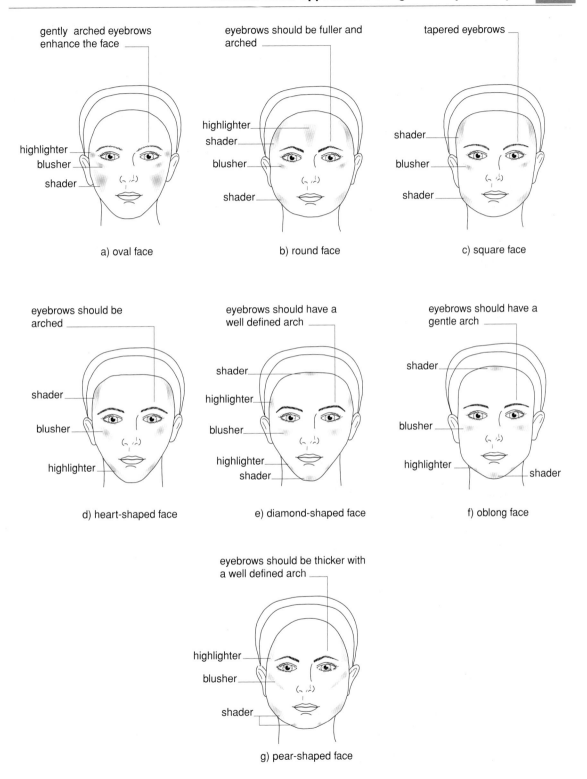

Figure 5.5 Highlighter, blusher and shader are used in corrective make-up

PREPARATION OF THE TREATMENT AREA

It is important to ensure the trolley and work station are prepared prior to the client's arrival. Your work station should be equipped with:

- cleansing, toning and moisturising mediums – a selection should be available to accommodate the findings of the skin analysis
- corrective products – green tinted moisturiser, concealer products
- foundations – a selection of shades
- contour cosmetics – highlighters, shaders, blushers
- eyeshadows – a selection of colours with both matt and pearlised finish
- mascaras – block-type with disposable wands
- false lashes – individual and strip lashes
- brow cosmetics
- lip cosmetics.

In addition you will need:

- cotton wool and cotton wool buds
- tissues
- spatulas
- a selection of bowls
- headband
- mirror
- a covered waste receptacle
- client treatment plan or record card.

All tools and equipment should be sterilised in the appropriate way (see page 21) and should not be brought to the trolley until you are ready to use them.

The client should be comfortably positioned on the couch or make-up chair. The client should be in an **elevated** position and should not be lying flat for make-up application. It is important that the effects of gravity on the facial features are considered. The hair and clothes should be protected. The therapist can be either seated or standing, depending on the working height of the couch or chair. At least 20 minutes should be allowed for make-up application in the treatment schedule.

PREPARATION OF THE SKIN

The skin must be clean and free from grease, stale make-up and cleansing products. Once the skin is cleansed, a suitable moisturiser should be applied to the face and neck. (See page 171 for more detail on cleansing and moisturising.)

> **NOTE!** It can be useful to blot with a tissue after applying moisturiser. This allows the foundation to be applied evenly.

Element 5.3

Apply make-up to meet client requirements

FOUNDATIONS

The right foundation is the basis of a successful make-up. Although it is not essential, it does provide the ideal surface to receive other cosmetics. A good foundation will even out the complexion, correct any imperfections and act as a barrier between the skin and any atmospheric pollution. Many foundations contain sunscreens to protect the skin from the damaging effects of ultra-violet light.

Selecting the right foundation

Factors to consider:

1. skin type
2. coverage
3. skin colour
4. lifestyle
5. occasion
6. expense
7. age.

Types of foundation

Foundations are available in many forms, the most common types being **creams**, **all-in-ones**, **liquids**, **cakes** and **gels**.

Type of foundation	Method of application
Creams – originally cream foundations were colour free, oil-in-water emulsions known as vanishing creams. Modern foundations are tinted and are usually oil-in-water emulsions containing mineral oil and ceresin wax. Colours range from the palest tones through to rich dark brown, thus providing a foundation colour to suit all skin colours. The cream may be coloured by the use of inorganic pigments such as iron oxides. The inclusion of titanium dioxide in the formulation produces a more opaque cream, increasing the covering power.	The foundation is removed from the container using a spatula and a small amount is placed on the back of the therapists hand or onto a palette. It can then be applied with fingertips using a light effleurage movement producing an even film over the skin.

Type of foundation	Method of application
All-in-one – this type of product is a mixture of cream foundation and face powder, which produces a foundation with a matt finish. The products are gaining in popularity, as they dispense with the need for separate foundation and powder.	These products are usually applied with the use of a facial wedge or sponge. A small amount of the product is placed onto the back of the therapist's hand or onto a palette. The foundation is then dotted using fingertips to one area of the face at a time and blended with the sponge.
Liquid – these contain similar ingredients to creams, but with a higher proportion of water. Some liquids are oil free, containing clay to thicken and hold the pigment in an alcohol or water base.	Liquid foundations should be gently agitated prior to use to disperse the pigments evenly through the formulation. The product may then be applied into the palm of the non-working hand of the therapist or onto a palette. Fingertip application is better for this product as moistened sponges can remove rather than apply. It is important to let this product dry before proceeding to the next stage.
Cake – cake foundations are usually emulsions containing mineral oils, wax, powder and pigments which are dried. The product is then powdered and compressed into cake form. Cake foundations give dense cover and can be used for correcting or concealing blemishes. This formulation is also used for **concealers**.	Cake foundations should be applied with a moistened sponge, slowly building up to the required finish.
Gels – these foundations produce a glossy film, often used to produce a tanned look. Gels have very little covering power therefore are unsuitable for less than perfect skins.	Care should be taken with their application. Do not dot all over the face as this can lead to irregular patches and staining. The gel sets quite quickly on application leaving a concentration of colour. Instead, a small amount should be dotted on one area at a time and blended in before applying elsewhere.

NOTE! Always check around hairline and jawline for demarcation lines. If in doubt blend around these areas with a clean moistened sponge.

Skin type and foundation

It is vital, when selecting a foundation, that the client's skin type is considered. If the wrong product is selected, the completed make-up may be poor and the effect may not be long-lasting. Moisturisers, whilst an essential element of the process, will only have a temporary effect. The skin will revert to type as the day progresses. If the right product is selected and it is applied correctly, foundation should last throughout the day, should not change colour or need to be reapplied.

Skin Type	Choice of Foundation
Dry	Cream or Moisturising Liquid
Mature	Cream or Moisturising Liquid
Sensitive	Hypo-allergenic liquid or cream
Combination	Liquid or all-in-one
Oily	Liquid, water based, oil-free
Blemished/Acne	Oil-free liquid which is medicated

When selecting a foundation, you should aim to match the colour as closely to the natural skin colour as possible. If the colour is not selected with great care, the result may be an unattractive mask-like appearance. This is a particular problem when selecting foundations for black skins. Foundation is not always necessary on darker skins, if the colour is even. Instead, a light dusting of translucent powder should be used to take off any excess shine and to provide a good base for the rest of the make-up application. If foundation is used, then it should be selected on the basis of complementing the lightest tones of the skin. Foundation should always be tested on the face, NOT the back of the hand. The skin on the hand is very different in both colour and texture and will not show the true effect of the product.

> **NOTE!** There may be an erythema present after cleansing, particularly on clients with a sensitive skin condition. This condition may be temporary and must be considered when making your foundation selection.

Colour suggestions

Skin Tones	Foundation Tones
Fair/pale, translucent skins	Light ivory, porcelain, apricot and peach tones
Medium skin	Beige and honey tones for medium light skin Warm apricots and olive for medium dark skin
Dark skin	Beige, bronze and olive tones

Skin Tones	Foundation Tones
Vascular complexions	Always use green corrective products to tone down redness Use beige and olive tones
Sallow skin	Pink, beige or tawny tones
Pigmented skin	Areas of pigmentation should be covered with camouflage cream before foundation is used

Hints

1. Choose a foundation to suit skin type and colour.
2. Choose a foundation as near to the natural skin colour as possible.
3. On dark skins select a product nearest to the lightest skin tone.
4. To reduce a florid skin apply green corrective cream before the foundation.
5. To brighten a sallow skin apply lilac corrective cream.
6. Apply foundation with a dampened make-up sponge or fingertips.
7. Apply foundation to small areas at a time and blend well.
8. If the under-eye area is very lined, mix a little moisturiser with the foundation and blend in up to the base of the lashes.

FACE POWDERS

Face powders can be either translucent (loose) or highly pigmented (usually compressed). They work in very different ways.

Translucent powder

Translucent powder is extra fine and filtered. It allows light to diffuse through without changing the underlying skin colour. The foundation should always be followed by application of loose powder. Translucent powder is designed to set the make-up but not to change the colour. Translucent powders enhance the foundation and tone down shine.

Compressed powder

Compressed powders offer dense coverage and, therefore, are restricted to corrective work or for make-up 'touch-ups'. The use of traditional compressed powder has decreased. This is due in part to the introduction of refined compressed foundations which offer good coverage with a velvety finish all from one product.

> **NOTE!** A good face powder should be easy to apply, be smooth on the skin and allow the colour of the foundation to be seen, without changing the base colour. Some powders can be worn without a base and can be used to give a glow to the skin, particularly on black or dark skins.

The main constituent of powder is **talc** which gives slip, translucency and covering power. Metallic particles may be added to give a pearly look. They should be used with caution. They can make the skin look moist especially when photographed, as the metallic particles reflect light. This type of powder is particularly effective for evening wear and could easily be added to adapt day make-up for evening.

Corrective effects of face powders
Translucent
Usually colourless and will not alter the desired effect of the make-up.

Green
As with tinted moisturisers, this coloured powder can be used under normal face powder to tone down a florid or red skin. It should be used sparingly, especially on the nose and cheek areas.

Lilac/Pale Pink
This can liven sallow skins. It should be used under normal face powder.

White/Pearly Powder
It may be used as a highlighter to enhance facial features.

Face powder application
A small amount of loose powder should be taken from the container using a clean spatula. The powder should be placed on to a tissue in the therapist's hand. A clean, sterile powder puff or ball of cotton wool should be dipped into the powder and the excess tapped off. A light twisting motion should be used to apply the product. A large headed powder brush should then be employed to dust away the excess powder from the face. This should be done with light upward and downward movements and will create a velvety finish to the skin.

> **NOTE!** Always apply a light dusting of powder to the lips and eyelids. This will help the eye and lip cosmetics respectively adhere to the area.

Hints
1. Always use loose powder.
2. **Never** apply powder which is darker than the foundation.
3. Apply sparingly if the skin is excessively dry or if the under-eye area is wrinkled.
4. If there is a lot of facial hair, powder should be avoided.

CONTOUR COSMETICS

Contour cosmetics comprise of three main types: blusher or rouge, highlighter and shader. They can be used to accentuate and diminish features or can be used to add colour and warmth.

Shading and highlighting can be done effectively on light or darker skins. However, shading will be less prominent on darker skins whilst highlighting will be more obvious.

Blusher or rouge

Blusher and rouge have the same function. Blusher is the modern name for rouge. It is designed to add colour to the cheek area, simulating a 'natural' cheek colour or adding warmth. It can be in cream or powder form and the colours available vary from very pale pinks through to brick reds and dark browns. Powder blusher is applied over foundation and after the powder has been applied. Cream blusher is usually applied after the foundation but before the powder.

Application

A small amount of powder blusher should be taken up onto a blusher brush. The excess should be tapped off over the back of the hand. The application should proceed using an inverted triangle as a template shape. Application should start from below the centre of the eye working up to the top of the ear. The application should not start any lower than below the centre of the client's eye. Without reloading the brush, small strokes gradually fanning out back up the cheekbone should be applied.

> **NOTE!** Do not exceed application below the centre of the client's eye. This can make the application look unnatural and can lead to the cheek having a 'sucked in' appearance.

Highlighters

Highlighters are used to enhance positive features. They are usually light colours: beiges and pinks through to white. Some may have pearlised or iridescent finishes and they can be cream or powder based. They are commonly used to accentuate the eyelids, under the eyebrow or across the cheekbone. Less common but equally effective, is the application of highlighter to the cupids bow on the lips to accentuate the pout. On darker skins, highlighting can be used to great effect. Areas of the face can be brought into prominence and interesting planes given to the features. Highlighting is particularly effective when used to slim and straighten the centre of the nose and give definition to the cheekbones.

Shaders

Shaders, as a range of corrective products, have been replaced with blushers and foundations. The **concept** of shading, however, is still very important. The effect of shading is to reduce or diminish a particular facial feature. Dark pink, tawny or brown shades are used and always have a matt finish. Shading is usually only used on darker skins to give depth to a rounded face around the lower cheek area. The wide colour range of foundations and blushers provides alternatives to a traditional shading product. Two foundations of contrasting colour can provide a natural shading effect.

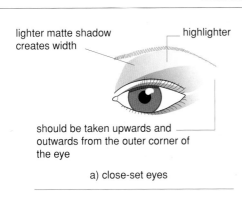

lighter matte shadow creates width

highlighter

should be taken upwards and outwards from the outer corner of the eye

a) close-set eyes

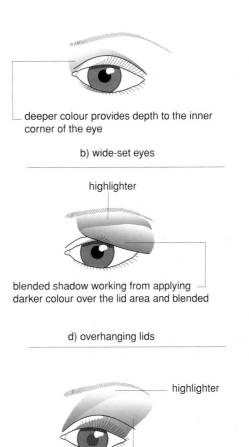

deeper colour provides depth to the inner corner of the eye

b) wide-set eyes

highlighter

blended shadow working from applying darker colour over the lid area and blended

d) overhanging lids

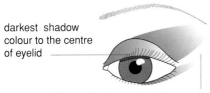

darkest shadow colour to the centre of eyelid

lift eyeshadow and eyeliner application beyond outer corner of eye

c) round or prominent eyes

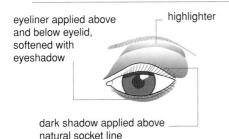

eyeliner applied above and below eyelid, softened with eyeshadow

highlighter

dark shadow applied above natural socket line

e) small or deep-set eyes

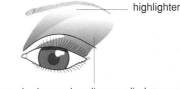

highlighter

dark eye shadow and eyeliner applied upwards and outwards to lift eye

f) downward slanting eyes

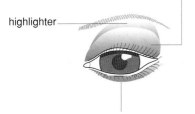

darken the socket line extending above natural socket line, blended into highlighter

highlighter

eyeliner applied to lower lash line and softened with eyeshadow

g) narrow eyes

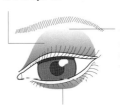

shading above the natural socket line gives depth to the eyelids

lighter matte eyeshadow blended across the eye socket gives depth and fullness to the eyes

eyeliner and eyeshadow applied to the lower lash line widens and enlarges

h) oriental eyes

Figure 5.6 Corrective eye make-up

Hints

1. All cream products should be applied **before** the powder. Powder products should be applied **after** the powder.
2. Blusher should always be kept high on the face and never applied to the centre plains of the cheeks.
3. Do not apply blusher too near to the nose or eyes.
4. The effect of contour products should be subtle and natural.
5. Check the application on completion to ensure it is symmetrical. Balance can also be achieved by applying a touch of colour at the temples.
6. Blend contour cosmetics carefully to ensure there is no demarcation line.

CONCEALERS

These are specially formulated to disguise minor imperfections and blemishes. They are cream based and are available in a range of flesh tones. These products are usually applied with a brush, cotton wool bud or fingertips, and normally before the foundation is applied.

Hints

1. The use of a white concealer cream is particularly effective in disguising dark circles under the eye.
2. Clients with high colouring or broken capillaries (couperose skin) could have a green tinted cream applied to the area. This reduces the redness.
3. Minor blemishes can be masked with concealer or lighter foundation using a brush.

NOTE! Use concealer products sparingly.

EYESHADOW

The eye shadow is one of the most important aspects of a good make-up. The shape of the eyes can be flattered or altered with an expert application of eyeshadow products. The choice of eyeshadow available now is overwhelming and care must be taken to discuss with the client their preferences and needs. If the make-up is for a special occasion, find out more about the function and explore the colour of the outfit to be worn. Ascertain the type of function – a different effect will be required for a wedding, party or a job interview. The application techniques for the products already covered are largely the same whichever type of function the client will be attending. The eye make-up application, however, will differ. The main function of eyeshadow is to accentuate the eyes and to make them look brighter. On a darker skin the eyes will need to be given added definition by emphasising the eyelashes as well as the eyelids. Eyeshadows are available in **powder, cream, gel** and **liquid** forms. They may have a matt finish, may contain metallic particles or have an iridescent effect.

Type of eyeshadow	Method of application
Powder eyeshadow – this is the type most commonly used. They are usually presented in a compressed cake, loose in a pot or in stick form. They are formulated in a similar way to cake products, but with stronger colour pigments added. Powder eyeshadow is very popular, but its staying power is limited unless foundation is used. Loose powders can irritate the eye, particularly if powdered metals are contained in the products. Clients with contact lenses should use compressed powders to prevent particles of powder entering the eye. A range of products has been designed to suit the needs of contact lens wearers and this could be a consideration when selecting a suitable retail range in the salon	A small amount of colour should be taken onto a sterilised eyeshadow brush. The excess should be tapped off over the back of the hand. The product should be applied to the closed eye according to the desired effect. A clean tissue should be placed under the eye to catch any loose particles and to prevent the therapist's hand coming into contact with the prepared 'canvas'.
Cream eyeshadow – cream eyeshadows are not as popular as the powder varieties. Their staying power is quite poor and it is difficult to prevent creasing in the socket line. If the client does prefer cream eyeshadow, it is important to apply a light dusting of powder over the eyeshadow to help it to set.	Cream eyeshadows can be applied with the fingertips or with a moistened sponge tipped applicator. A light dusting of powder should be applied to facilitate setting.
Gel or liquid eyeshadow – this type of eyeshadow has seen an increase in popularity. The effect created can enhance the eyes and the same product can also be used on the lips. They tend to give gloss rather than depth of colour. Several coats may be required to give adequate coverage.	These products can be applied with fingertips or with a small eyeshadow brush.

Corrective eye make-up
Hints

1. Cream eyeshadow must be applied before face powder.
2. Gel and powder eyeshadow are applied after powder.
3. Ascertain the function or effect required and explore colour themes.
4. Do not apply highlighter to loose, crepey (thin, wrinkled) lids.
5. Introduce a small amount of blue to the base of the lashes. This will brighten the whites of the eyes.
6. Take care to avoid contact between the client's face and your hand by placing a tissue underneath the hand.
7. Where there are dark circles under the eyes, concealer may be applied to lighten the effect.

EYELINER

Eyeliner is available in **liquid**, **pencil** or **cake** formulations. It is probably the most difficult cosmetic to apply, but once the technique is mastered it can add real definition to the eye. It can be used to encircle the eye lids or can be used on the outer edges of the lids only. The softer, non-setting formulations such as cake or pencil can be smudged using a sponge tipped applicator or a cotton wool bud. This gives a softer definition to the eyelid.

Liquid
This is used to give a definite line. Liquid liners are applied with a very fine brush for accuracy.

Pencil
Pencil liners should be sharpened before use on each new client. They can be applied in a hard line and then blended to soften the line depending upon the desired effect. Kohl also is available in pencil form and is soft and waxy in texture. It can be quite difficult to control because of its composition and the effect of the body heat on the waxes.

Cake
Cake liner is applied with a wet fine brush. It is similar to eyeshadows in composition and can be smudged once dry for a softer effect.

MASCARA

Mascara is used to give definition to the eyes by thickening and darkening the lashes. There are two types of mascara: **cake** and **liquid**.

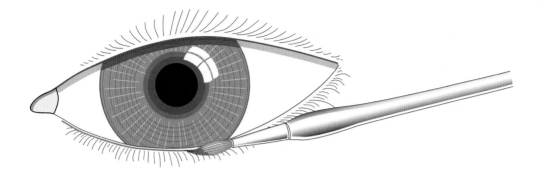

application of eyeliner

Figure 5.7 Application of eyeliner

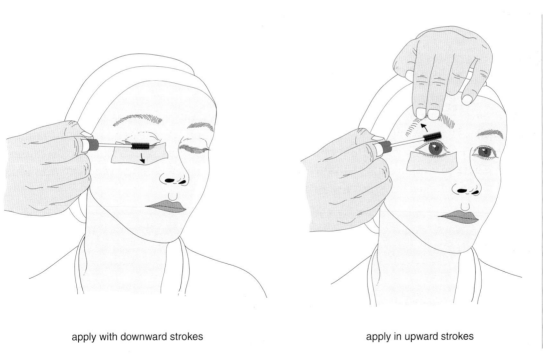

apply with downward strokes   apply in upward strokes

Figure 5.8 Applying mascara

Cake

This is applied with a moistened disposable brush. Cake mascaras are made from waxes and pigments in a soap base. The moisture from the brush creates the formation of an emulsion on the surface of the cake. The brush takes the emulsion up and it can be applied to the lashes.

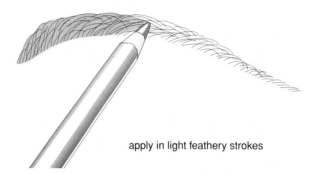

apply in light feathery strokes

Figure 5.9 Using an eyebrow pencil

Liquid

Liquid mascaras are available with a wide range of functions: waterproof, smudgeproof, hypoallergenic, lash lengthening, thickening, protein enriched. Colour pigments and resins are contained in a base of water or alcohol and water with castor oil to prevent the mascara from becoming brittle. Filaments of rayon or nylon can be used to build and 'extend' lashes. Mascaras that contain such filaments should not be used on contact lens wearers as the filaments can irritate the eye. These mascaras come with their own applicator wand within the product and should not be used in the salon as there is a risk of cross infection.

> **NOTE!** Always wipe over the lashes with a mild tonic solution before starting the make-up. This will ensure the lashes are completely grease free.

Application

1. Curl the lashes prior to mascara application if required.
2. Apply to lower lashes first, thus enabling the client to look upwards without fear of marking the brow area with damp mascara.
3. Place a tissue under the lower lashes.
4. Life the skin of the eyelids from underneath the brow when applying to the upper lashes.
5. Build up in fine coats, allowing each one to dry.
6. Separate using an eyelash comb if necessary.

> **NOTE!** Always use individual disposable applicator wands for each client to prevent cross infection.

Hints

1. If the client's eyes water, gently blot corner of eye with a soft tissue.
2. Don't apply to lower lashes if the skin is crepey.
3. Ensure the client is advised of the type of product used and the method or product to be used for removal, especially important for waterproof products.
4. Application of a light dusting of powder will help to thicken the lashes and increase adhesion of the mascara.

EYEBROW PENCILS

These are available in a range of hair colours: grey, brown and black.

They should be applied in light feathery strokes not in hard defined lines. They are used to add definition to the eyebrow area and can also be used in corrective work to balance or to infill missing brows.

Application

1. The brows should be brushed into shape before applying the pencil.
2. When applying, aim to create the appearance of natural hair growth by using light feathery strokes and brushing through after application to soften the effect.

Hints

1. A light application of a softer shade of eyeshadow can be used to good effect, if definition rather than correction is required.
2. Brush through brows after cosmetic application to soften effect.

LIP COSMETICS

Lip cosmetics are available in **pots**, **sticks** and **pencils**. They are each used to define, enhance and balance the lip shape. The main ingredients of lip products are oils, fats and waxes.

Lipstick

This has a high percentage of wax, which gives it its stiffened form. Lipsticks will vary in terms of their staying power and the choice of product will depend upon the finished effect required. When selecting lipstick for a darker skin, consideration should be given to the natural colour tones of the lips. It may be necessary to even the lip tone using a foundation or corrective product prior to application. A number of products claim to stay on all day. These products can be very drying and can also stain the lips. Softening ingredients such as petroleum jelly or mineral oil are also included in varying amounts depending on the formulation.

Gloss

This is usually formulated with a high grease content. Gloss can be clear or pigmented and is not durable. It should not be used on large lips as it will accentuate them. The introduction of a gel based gloss has brought increased durability. This product may also be used on the eyes.

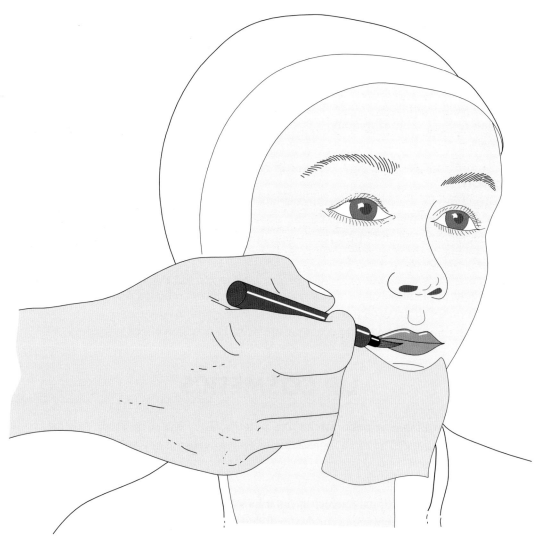

Figure 5.10 Applying lipstick with a brush

Pencil

This is used for outlining the lips. Pencils are difficult to sterilise and therefore must be sharpened prior to every use. They are formulated with a high proportion of hard waxes. Pencils are good for corrective lip work because they can be used to balance and even alter the alignment of the lips.

Application

1. If using a pencil, outline evenly the line of the lip.
2. If using lipstick, gently scrape a small amount of the chosen colour onto a clean palette or spatula and using a clean, sterilised lip brush, apply a clear outline to the lips. Then fill in the lips evenly with colour.
3. Outline the lips from the sides to the centre with the lips slightly apart to allow application into the corners of the mouth.
4. Protect the make-up by using a tissue on the client's chin to support the hand.
5. Blot after the first application and reapply. This prolongs the duration of the application.

Hints

1. Apply lipgloss over the lip colour for fashion or evening wear.
2. Avoid using blueish tones on sallow skin.
3. For uneven lip tones, even out using foundation or concealer prior to applying lip colour.
4. Avoid over use of lip gloss on large lips.

> **NOTE!** It is particularly important to keep accurate records of the selected make-up products and application method. These details must be entered on the client's treatment plan or record card for easy retrieval of data, continuity of future treatments and for marketing opportunities.

GENERAL PROCEDURE FOR MAKE-UP APPLICATION

1. Prepare client for make-up.
2. Check for contraindications.
3. Remove make-up brushes and sponges from the steriliser.
4. Conduct consultation with the client.
5. Select a foundation to suit the client's skin colour and type (see page 119).
6. Apply concealer if required.
7. Using a dampened cosmetic sponge, apply the foundation to the face. Take care to avoid the hairline and check for demarcation lines.
8. Place a small amount of loose powder into your tissue-lined palm. Using a dry piece of cotton wool or a sterilised powder puff, take up a small amount of powder. Lightly twist the powder into the foundation. Do not rub.
9. Select a large powder brush and sweep away any excess powder. Use upward and downward strokes to ensure that the fine facial hairs are lifted away from the skin. If you select a cream blusher this should be applied prior to the powder.
10. Apply blusher (see page 122).
11. Apply eyeshadows (see page 124).
12. Apply eyeliner (see page 126).
13. Apply mascara using disposable sterilised wands (see page 128).
14. Apply lipliner (see page 130).
15. Take a small amount of the selected lipstick onto a spatula and apply using a sterilised lipbrush, blot and reapply.
16. Check overall effect for balance.
17. Remove hair covering and tidy client's hair.
18. Show client the finished result.

SELF ASSESSMENT TEST

1. What corrective cosmetics would you use on a client with a sallow skin?
2. How could a day make-up be adapted for evening wear?
3. What steps should you take to avoid the risk of cross infection when using mascara?
4. List three reasons for keeping accurate records of clients' make-up.
5. What considerations should be given when selecting lip cosmetics for a black skin?

Activity

1 Collect pictures and photographs from magazines and other sources which have interesting make-up designs. Examine your cuttings and analyse technique. Look carefully at use of colour and continuation, and contrast of theme. Examine the use of accessories and backdrops. Put the pictures into a scrapbook and keep adding to it for future reference. This will become one of your most precious resources!

2 Experiment with different make-up colours and application techniques and produce a series of photographs. Include evidence of corrective work. These will be useful for your portfolio of evidence and will also be of value to demonstrate your abilities to prospective employers.

KEY SKILLS TASK FOR UNITS 5, 6, 7, 8 AND 9

Assess clients for treatment and prepare a treatment plan

1. Collect information to show that you have carried out consultations with different clients for a range of treatments. This could include:
   - client feedback in your diary or log
   - observation records by your beauty therapy assessor
   - client record cards and treatment plans.

   You will need to think about the following range of treatments:
   - Make-up – Unit 5
   - Facial treatments – Unit 6
   - Waxing and lightening hair – Unit 7
   - Lash and brow treatments – Unit 8
   - Manicure and Pedicure – Unit 9

2. Choose two clients, one of whom should be new to you, and write a summary on how you carried out the consultation. Include examples of the questions you asked and what information you gained from the questioning.

3. Calculate the cost of a course of:
   - six pedicure treatments
   - four lash tints.

   Use your salon price list to make the calculation and take account of VAT.

Application of number

Element 1 Collect and record data

Evidence Calculating the cost of treatments to include VAT

Problem solving
Element 1 Used established procedures to clarify routine problems

Evidence Make decisions about contraindications and appropriate treatment based on information gained from the client

Communication
Element 1 Take part in discussion

Evidence Discussion with a client during the consultation

Element 2 Produce written material

Evidence Produce a range of completed record cards and treatment plans

Element 4 Read and respond to written material

Evidence Using the ongoing information contained in record cards to adapt treatment plans

Working with others
Element 1 Identify collective goals

Evidence Treatment plan agreed with the client

Element 2 Work to collective goals

Evidence Written feedback provided by clients in your log/diary or on the record card on the success of the series of treatments

UNIT 6

Improve facial skin condition

In this unit you will learn about:

- bones of the head, neck and shoulders
- muscles of the head and neck
- blood supply to the head and neck
- lymph nodes of the head and neck
- nerve supply to the head and neck
- assessing client skin type
- assessing client skin type
- preparing the treatment area effectively and hygienically
- cleansing
- massaging the client's face, neck and shoulders
- advising on facial aftercare.

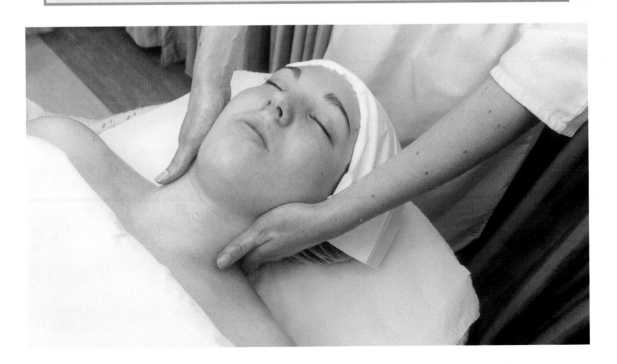

INTRODUCTION

The development of a suitable treatment plan will hinge upon accurate analysis of the skin. It is also important to discuss client needs and expectations, to ensure they are realistic and can be met.

This unit will help you to put together appropriate treatments to improve the client's skin condition. It will help you to recognise **contraindications** (conditions which prohibit treatment), **contra-actions** (reactions to treatment) and **indications** (where conditions will respond to treatment) to treatment through effective assessment of skin and the subsequent preparation of a treatment plan.

BONES OF THE HEAD, NECK AND SHOULDER

Bones are hard structures which link together to form the skeleton. It is this which gives the body shape and support. Where two bones come together a joint is formed.

Functions of the skeleton

1. shape and support
2. protection
3. production of blood cells
4. calcium storage
5. muscle and tendon attachment
6. movement and locomotion.

The skeleton is made up of two type of tissue: **cartilage** and **bone**. Cartilage is less rigid than bone and slightly elastic. It is found on the articulating surfaces of bones, in other words at movable joints. Bone is a rigid structure composed of water, organic matter and inorganic salts, chiefly calcium phosphate. Bones are living structures, so they have a blood and nerve supply and are influenced by changes in the diet, hormone levels and any stresses that they are exposed to, such as injury or over use.

The blood supply running through the bones provides nutrients which are stored or removed depending on the demands of the body. The blood brings the required nutrients and oxygen necessary for red blood cell formation which occurs in the bone marrow of the long bones.

THE SKULL

The bones of the skull are divided into two groups: the cranial bones and the facial bones.

The cranium

There are eight bones which form a box-like structure to protect the brain; this box is called the cranium. There are:

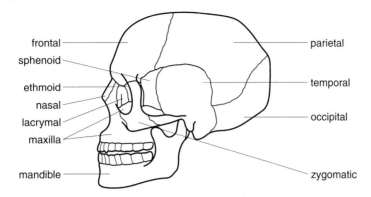

Figure 6.1 A skull viewed from the side

- one **occipital** bone forming the back of the cranium
- two **parietal** bones forming the top, back part of the cranium
- one **frontal** bone forming the top, front part of the cranium, the forehead and the upper part of the eye sockets
- two **temporal** bones forming the sides of the cranium, above and around the ears
- one **sphenoid** bone forming the base of the cranium with wings on either side forming the temples
- one **ethmoid** bone lying between the frontal and sphenoid bones forming the roof of the nasal cavities.

The face

There are 14 bones forming the facial structure and these are largely responsible for the face shape. There are:

- two **zygomatic** bones forming the cheekbones
- two **maxillae** bones forming the upper jaw, side walls of the nose and front of the hard palate – the upper teeth are embedded in the maxillae
- two **palatine** bones forming the roof of the mouth and part of the sides of the nose
- two **lacrimal** bones forming the inner sides of the eye sockets
- two **nasal** bones forming the bridge of the nose
- two **turbinate** bones forming the nasal passages inside the nose
- one **vomer** bone also forming the nasal passages
- one **mandible** bone forming the lower jaw – the lower teeth are embedded in the mandible.

Most of the bones of the skull form **fixed joints**, called **sutures**. The only free-moving joint is that between the mandible and the temporal bones which allows the lower jaw to move up and down, as in chewing.

THE NECK

The neck forms part of the **vertebral column** which is a series of irregular shaped bones stacked on top of each other to form a column. Each **vertebra** is separated from the one above and below it by a disc of cartilage which prevents the bones rubbing against each other and acts as a cushion or shock absorber for stress administered from the upper body to the lower or vice versa. The bones are named after the area in which they are situated, hence the neck bones are called the **cervical vertebrae** and there are seven of them in total. The diagram below shows their relationship with the skull and the shoulder.

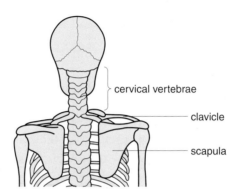

Figure 6.2 Bones of the neck and shoulder viewed from behind

The upper two vertebrae nearest the skull are specialised and have a different shape to the others. The top vertebrae is attached to the underneath of the **sphenoid** bone and has a hole through which passes a peg-like structure of the second vertebrae. This arrangement forms a special joint called a **pivot** joint that allows rotation of the head.

THE SHOULDER

The shoulder is a complicated, free-moving joint situated at the top of the arm and is made up of the **clavicle** and **scapula** bones.

The clavicle

Commonly known as the **collarbone**, this forms an s-shape from the breastbone to the shoulder, where joints are formed at both ends.

The scapula

The scapula is a flat bone of triangular shape lying in the upper back, commonly known as the **shoulder blade**. It forms a loose joint at the shoulder with the clavicle and relies on strong ligament and muscle attachment for its stability.

The diagram in Figure 6.3 shows the location of these bones and their relationship with the neck and skull.

SELF ASSESSMENT TEST
1. Name five functions of the skeleton.
2. The shoulder is made up of which bones?
3. What is the correct name for the neck bones?
4. What is the correct name for the cheekbones?
5. Which bones make up the cranium?
6. What is the function of the cranium?
7. What is the correct name for the lower jaw?
8. Which bones form the eye sockets?
9. Which bones have the upper and lower teeth embedded in them?
10. Where can the only free-moving joint be found in the skull?

MUSCLES OF THE FACE, NECK AND SHOULDER

Muscle is a special type of tissue that is able to contract. When it does so the muscle becomes shorter and fatter and feels hard to the touch. There are three types of muscle tissue:
- **voluntary muscle** is tissue which brings about movement. This type of muscle tissue is also called **skeletal muscle** as it is attached to the bones or **striped muscle** as, when viewed under a microscope, bands of light and dark can be seen.
- **involuntary muscle**, found in the digestive tract and blood vessels.
- **cardiac muscle** found only in the heart.

Voluntary muscle contraction is brought about by a series of events. Firstly, the central nervous system, the brain and spinal cord, send a message in the form of an electrical impulse along a **motor nerve** to the muscle. When it reaches the muscle the motor nerve attaches to the muscle fibres at the **motor point**. It divides so that each muscle fibre is connected by at least one nerve fibre. The message is passed from the nerve to the muscle fibres and the muscle contracts.

Movement is brought about by the ends of the muscles being connected to bones across a joint, the movement taking place at the joint. In the face, the muscles can be connected to bone at one end and skin at the other, or in some cases skin at both ends and along its entire length.

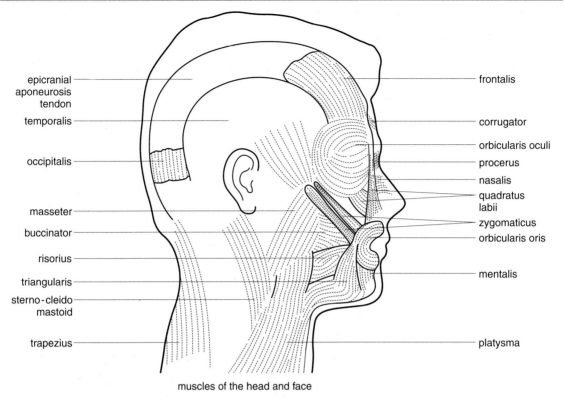

epicranial aponeurosis tendon		frontalis
temporalis		corrugator
		orbicularis oculi
occipitalis		procerus
		nasalis
		quadratus labii
masseter		zygomaticus
buccinator		orbicularis oris
risorius		
triangularis		mentalis
sterno-cleido mastoid		
trapezius		platysma

muscles of the head and face

Figure 6.3 Muscles of the face viewed from the side

MUSCLES OF THE FACE

Name of muscle	Position	Action
The occipitalis	found at the back of the head, attached to the occipital bone and the skin of the scalp	to move the scalp
The orbicularis oris	a circular muscle surrounding the mouth and its fibres occupy the entire width of the lips	closes or narrows the lips, used to press the lips against the teeth and to purse the lips as in whistling
The orbicularis oculi	surrounds the opening of the eye socket, attached to the bones at its outer edge and the skin of the upper and lower eyelids at the inner edge	to close the eyes as in sleeping, winking and blinking, also used when squinting

Name of muscle	Position	Action
The buccinator	the main muscle of the cheek – it is attached to both the upper and lower jaw and forms a muscular plate which fills the gap between them	its function is to keep the cheek stretched during all phases of opening and closing the mouth, also used to compress the cheeks, when blowing up a balloon or playing the trumpet, for example
The masseter	this muscle is closest to the surface, and stretches from the cheekbone to the lower jaw	it lifts the lower jaw, closing the jaw and exerting pressure on the teeth, used when chewing
The risorius	this muscle lies above the buccinator and is attached to the cheekbone at one end and the skin of the corner of the mouth at the other	it pulls the corner of the mouth sideways and upwards to create a grinning expression
The zygomaticus	lies in the inner cheek by the nose, from the zygomatic bone to the corners of the mouth	takes the corners of the mouth upward and laterally assisting the risorius muscle
The quadratus labii superioris	towards the inner cheek beside the nose, stretching from the upper jaw to the skin of the corners of the mouth and the upper lip	raises the upper lip and corner of the mouth to create a snarling expression
The nasalis	sides of the nose attached to the maxillae bones and the nostrils	dilates and compresses the nostril openings
The triangularis	a triangular shaped muscle under the corners of the mouth, stretching from the lower jaw to the skin and muscles of the corners of the mouth	draws down the corners of the mouth, creating an expression of sadness
The mentalis	located at the point of the chin, it is attached to the lower jaw and the skin of the lower lip	it lifts and wrinkles the skin of the chin and turns the lower lip outwards creating a pouting expression
The frontalis	across the width of the forehead, attached to the skin of the eyebrows and the frontal bone at the hairline	wrinkles the forehead and raises eyebrows, creating a surprised expression

Name of muscle	Position	Action
The corrugator	in between the eyebrows, attached to the frontalis muscle and the inner edge of the eyebrow	brings the eyebrows together creating a frowning expression
The procerus	in between the eyebrows, attached to the nasal bones and the frontalis muscle	draws the eyebrows inwards creating a puzzled expression
The temporalis	around and behind the ear, stretching in front of the ear to the upper part of the lower jaw	raises the lower jaw when chewing

MUSCLES OF THE NECK AND SHOULDER

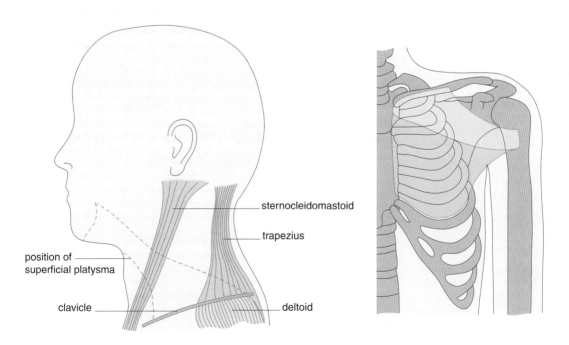

Figure 6.4 Muscles of the neck and shoulder

Name of muscle	Position	Action
The sternocleido-mastoid	powerful muscle lying obliquely across the side of the neck, from the collar and breast bones to the back of the ear	when the muscle on one side of the neck contracts, the head rotates to the opposite side, when both muscles are contracted together the chin is pulled down towards the chest
The platysma	extends down the front of the neck from the sides of the chin to the collar bones, either side of the throat	depresses the lower jaw and lip causing wrinkling in the skin of the neck especially when yawning
The trapezius	diamond shaped muscle at the upper back, neck and shoulder, stretches from the occipital bone of the skull and the vertebrae of the thorax to the scapula and outer end of the clavicle	raises the shoulder to the ear, holds the shoulder and scapula still during arm movements and pulls the head backwards
The pectoralis	in the chest below the clavicle, stretches from the sternum across the ribs to the humerus	brings the arm forward and across the chest, used in pushing
The deltoid	forms the cap of the shoulder, the front comes from the clavicle and back from the scapula, the two heads meet and attach to the humerus	the front part brings the arm forward, the back takes it backwards together they take the arm out sideways.

BLOOD SUPPLY TO THE FACE AND NECK

Blood is a liquid which travels inside vessels called:

- arteries
- arterioles
- veins
- venules
- capillaries.

The blood moves along these vessels due to the pumping action of the heart, which is made of a muscle tissue called **cardiac muscle**.

Blood itself is made up of a fluid called **plasma**, this being mostly water with salts and waste products dissolved in it. Floating in the plasma are **red** and **white blood cells**, **platelets** and **blood proteins** eg fibrinogen (which helps the blood to clot).

The functions of blood
1 Transport
- oxygen is carried from the lungs to all living tissues
- carbon dioxide is carried from the tissues to the lungs to be exhaled
- nutrients from the digestive system are carried to the tissues
- excess water is taken from the tissues to the kidneys for excretion
- waste products from cell activity are taken to the kidneys or skin for excretion
- hormones released from endocrine glands are carried to their target organs.

2 Defence
- white blood cells are taken to a site of injury to fight invading bacteria and so stop infection
- other white blood cells produce **antibodies** that fight diseases which have entered the blood stream
- blood proteins and platelets combine at the site of injury or damage to form a clot that plugs the wound preventing blood loss and the invasion of bacteria. The clot hardens to form a scab which protects the area while new tissue grows underneath.

3 Heat distribution and regulation
- body heat produced in the organs and muscles of the body is distributed around the body to maintain a temperature of 37°C.
- the dilation of the blood capillaries in the skin allows excess heat to be lost to the atmosphere. When the temperature of the body needs to be maintained, the blood capillaries constrict preventing blood nearing the surface of the skin.

Blood circulation
As mentioned previously, blood is moved along the vessels by the pumping action of the heart. The heart has four chambers: **right atrium**; **right ventricle**; **left atrium**; **left ventricle**. A wall separates the left and right sides and valves which open and close separate the top chambers from the bottom.

The valves allow blood to flow from the top atrium into the bottom ventricles. When the heart contracts or beats, the right side beats just before the left and this pushes blood out of the **ventricles** into the blood vessels. Other valves in the vessels prevent the blood from reversing back into the heart so that when it relaxes blood is drawn into the **atrium**. The vessels from the lower right ventricle carry blood to the lungs where it gives up carbon dioxide and takes on fresh oxygen. It then returns to the heart entering the top left atrium. The blood passes through the valve into the bottom left ventricle where it is pumped out along a large vessel called the **aorta** which supplies the whole body with blood. To complete the journey, blood returns from the areas of the body to the top right chamber to begin the cycle again.

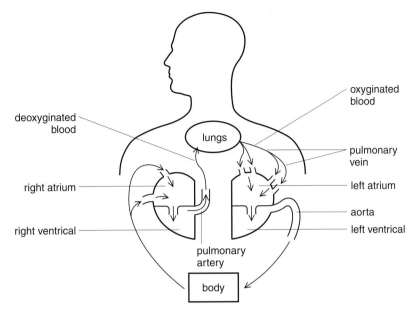

Figure 6.5 A simplified diagram to show blood circulation

Blood supply to the head and neck

Oxygenated blood leaves the heart through the aorta, this large vessel stretches upwards in front of the heart and then arches over to run down behind it. As it does so two smaller arteries branch off and travel upwards on either side of the neck. Once in the neck area they are called the **common carotid arteries** and as they near the head they divide to form the **external and internal carotid arteries**. At the level of the ear, the internal carotid disappears through a hole in the skull to supply blood to the brain and eyes. The external carotid artery splits further to supply blood to the skin and muscles of the face and scalp. There are three main branches called the **facial artery**, the **temporal artery** and the **occipital artery** and they supply blood to the areas after which they were named.

As arteries become smaller they are known as **arterioles**. These become smaller still until they are the thickness of a hair when they are known as **capillaries**. The walls of a capillary are very thin, just one cell thick. This allows the food and oxygen contained within the blood to be lost to the surrounding tissues and the waste products of cell activity to be collected by the blood. This process is called **capillary exchange**. Once this has happened the blood begins its journey back to the heart. The capillaries join to form small vessels called **venules**, which in turn join up to form **veins**. The veins returning the blood back to the heart from the head and neck are called the **internal and external jugular veins**. The former exiting the skull through a hole near the ear as before and the external jugular vein draining blood from the **facial**, **temporal** and **occipital veins**.

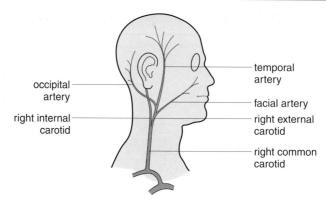

Figure 6.6 Arteries of the head and neck

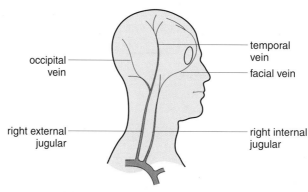

Figure 6.7 Veins of the head and neck

The internal and external jugular veins do not join together but run down the neck independently to join a large vein which eventually returns the blood to the heart.

SELF ASSESSMENT TEST
1. What is the name given to the fluid part of blood?
2. Name three main blood vessels.
3. Name the vessel that carries oxygenated blood away from the heart.
4. Name the vessel that carries deoxygenated blood back to the heart.
5. List the three functions of blood.
6. Name the two branches of the common carotid artery.
7. Name the three branches of the external carotid artery.
8. Name the vein that takes blood from the temple region.
9. Name the two veins that take deoxygenated blood away from the head.
10. What is the name given to the process by which waste products are swapped for food and oxygen in the tissues?

THE LYMPHATIC SYSTEM

The lymphatic system defends the body from infection and works as a waste disposal system. It consists of fine tubes or **lymph capillaries** present within the tissues. These collect the **tissue fluid** containing waste products, toxins and micro-organisms. Once inside the lymph capillaries the fluid is known as **lymph**. The composition of lymph is similar to that of blood plasma but it contains less blood proteins and food materials and more waste material. White blood cells are numerous in the lymph. The lymph capillaries join to form a network of vessels running alongside the blood vessels with the lymph travelling in the same direction as the venous flow, towards the heart. This is known as **lymph drainage**.

Lymph capillaries

These are fine, blind-ended tubes about the size of a human hair. They are present between the cells of all tissues but are found in large numbers in the areas of the body most likely to become infected or where micro-organisms can enter easily such as the toes, fingers, around the stomach and small intestine, the mouth, ears, eyes and nose.

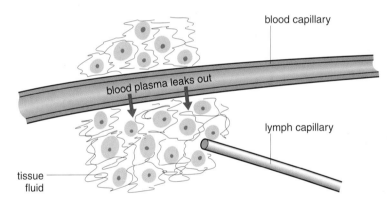

Figure 6.8 Tissue fluid leaks out of blood capillaries and into the surrounding tissues. It drains into lymph capillaries

Lymph vessels

The lymph capillaries form a network which join to form larger **lymph vessels**. These are similar to veins in structure and in the direction in which they run. They have thin, weak muscular walls and valves to prevent the backflow of lymph.

The lymphatic system relies on the pumping action of surrounding muscles to move the lymph along these vessels. As the muscles contract they become shorter and fatter which squeezes the lymph vessels and pushes the lymph along, the valves preventing its return. This causes a vacuum below the valve, which is filled from lymph further down the vessel. This reaction reoccurs as far as the lymph capillaries which causes more tissue fluid to be drawn into them.

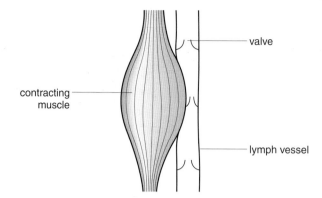

Figure 6.9 Muscle contraction squeezes fluid along the lymph vessels

Lymph nodes

Lymph nodes are areas where the lymph is cleansed by firstly being filtered and then by the action of special white blood cells present in the node. These cells destroy micro-organisms and other unwanted material so that when the lymph leaves the node it consists of mainly white blood cells and food materials. The nodes are found in groups in order for the lymph to be cleansed several times before being deposited back in the blood stream.

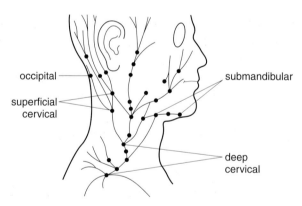

Figure 6.10 Lymph nodes of the head and neck

Lymph ducts

Once the lymph has been cleansed it travels along vessels to the chest area where it is deposited back into the blood stream through tubes called **lymph ducts**. Lymph collected from the right side of the head, chest and the right arm drains into the **right lymphatic duct** whilst lymph from the rest of the body drains into the **thoracic duct**. These ducts deposit the lymph into the subclavian veins.

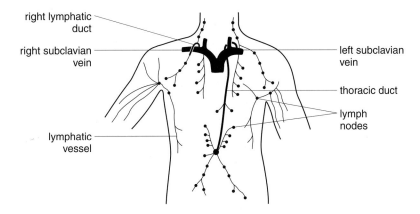

right lymphatic duct

right subclavian vein

left subclavian vein

thoracic duct

lymph nodes

lymphatic vessel

Figure 6.11 Lymph ducts

Factors affecting lymph drainage

1. **General blood circulation** – if the heart works well there will be good lymph drainage due to capillary exchange in the tissues, if not **oedema** (swelling) will occur.
2. **Exercise** – the action of the muscles on the lymph vessels speeds up lymph drainage and improves the performance of the heart.
3. **Massage** – Deep movements press on the lymph vessels forcing the lymph along them. These movements are always performed towards the heart, that is in the direction of lymph flow. See page 177 for further information on these massage techniques.

The effects of lymph drainage on skin and muscle tissue

Good lymph drainage benefits the function and appearance of the skin and enhances the performance of muscle tissue by improving the internal environment through the removal of waste material. The removal of the waste allows further capillary exchange to occur with the local blood capillaries, hence more food and oxygen is provided for the cells.

The functions of the lymphatic system

1. To fight infection.
2. To return food and proteins from the tissues to the blood circulatory system.
3. To transport white blood cells from the nodes to the blood circulatory system.
4. To transport fat from the small intestine to the liver.
5. To prevent oedema (swelling) by draining tissue fluid from the tissues.
6. To produce white blood cells (lymphocytes).

SELF ASSESSMENT TEST

Below are a list of statements. You are to decide whether they are true or false.

1. The lymphatic system takes waste products away from the tissues of the body. TRUE/FALSE
2. An important function of the white blood cells is to fight infection. TRUE/FALSE
3. The structure of a lymph vessel is similar to an artery. TRUE/FALSE
4. Lymph nodes produce white blood cells. TRUE/FALSE
5. Lymph capillaries have valves to prevent backflow of lymph. TRUE/FALSE
6. Lymph drainage is aided by the pumping action of muscles. TRUE/FALSE
7. Lymph drainage is aided by massage. TRUE/FALSE
8. Lymph nodes filter lymph to cleanse it. TRUE/FALSE
9. Lymph originates from blood plasma. TRUE/FALSE
10. Cleansed lymph is returned to the blood stream. TRUE/FALSE

THE NERVOUS SYSTEM

The nervous system consists of special cells called **neurones** that make up the **brain**, **spinal cord** and pairs of **nerves** and its function is to receive and transmit impulses or messages to and from organs and muscles. In doing so, the nervous system integrates and controls all the functions of the body.

The nerves of the head and neck

The fifth and seventh cranial nerves are responsible for the sensations and movement of the facial muscles.

The fifth cranial nerve or trigeminal nerve

This is mainly a sensory nerve carrying information to the brain from the skin of the face, the teeth and the membranes of the nose and mouth. There is also a motor branch to the muscles of mastication. The main branches are the mandibular, maxillary and ophthalmic branches.

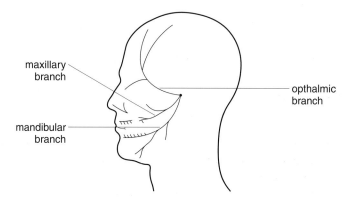

Figure 6.12 Branches of the fifth cranial or trigeminal nerve

The Mandibular Branch
- **Sensory** – for the teeth of lower jaw, membranes of mouth and cheeks, and the skin of the lower part of the face.
- **Motor** – to the masseter and temporalis (the muscles of chewing).

The Maxillary Branch
- **Sensory** – for the upper jaw, the skin on the temples, sides of forehead, and upper cheeks.

The Ophthalmic Branch
- **Sensory** – for tear glands, and the skin of forehead, nose and upper eyelids.

The seventh cranial nerve or facial nerve

This is mainly a motor nerve serving the muscles of facial expression, but has a small sensory branch for the sensation of taste from the front of the tongue. There are five main branches.

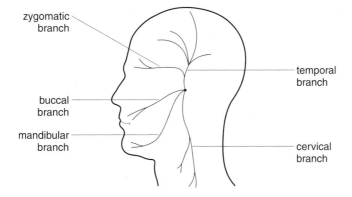

Figure 6.13 Branches of the seventh cranial or facial nerve

1. **The Temporal Branch**
   - **Motor** – leads to the muscles of the ear, the orbicularis oculi and the frontalis.
2. **The Zygomatic Branch**
   - **Motor** – leads to the orbicularis oculi.
3. **The Buccal Branch**
   - **Motor** – leads to the buccinator, the upper lip, and sides of the nose.
4. **The Mandibular Branch**
   - **Motor** – leads to the lower lip and the mentalis muscle.
   - **Sensory** – from the front of the tongue.
5. **The Cervical Branch**
   - **Motor** – leads to the platysma muscle in the neck.

> **NOTE!** The sternomastoid and the trapezius muscles are served by the 11th Cranial Nerve or Accessory Nerve

The nervous system is divided into two parts. These are the central and the peripheral systems.

The central nervous system (CNS)

The brain and the spinal cord make up the CNS. These important organs are protected by bone that completely surrounds them. In the case of the brain, it is the **cranium** and the spinal cord is protected by the **vertebrae** of the spine. From the brain and spinal cord come pairs of nerves that make up the peripheral nervous system.

The peripheral nervous system

There are 12 pairs of nerves from the brain called **cranial** nerves and 31 pairs from the spinal cord called **spinal nerves**. Each pair can contain either **motor** or **sensory** neurones or both.

- Sensory neurones take messages from the sense organs such as those in the skin to the central nervous system.
- Motor neurones take messages from the CNS to muscles or glands such as the sweat glands in the skin.

The autonomic nervous system

The autonomic nervous system is a specialised part of the peripheral nervous system and is **involuntary**, in other words under subconscious control. It is responsible for controlling involuntary actions of the body such as heart beat, breathing rate, pupil dilation and the involuntary muscles that make up the blood vessels and digestive tract. There are two parts:

1. **The Parasympathetic System** helps to create the conditions needed for rest, sleep and digestion.
2. **The Sympathetic System** works antagonistically with the parasympathetic system to create the conditions needed for physical activity. It works with the hormone **adrenaline** to prepare the body for 'fight or flight' and is responsible for the conditions associated with 'stress' in modern day living.

The effects of the autonomic system are summarised in the table below:

Part of body affected	Sympathetic	Parasympathetic
pupils	dilate	constrict
blood vessels	of digestive trace – constrict giving the feeling of 'butterflies' Of skeletal muscles – dilate Tone is increased in walls of larger vessels leading to high blood pressure	Of glands – dilate
heartbeat	quick and strong	slow and weak
breathing	quick and deep	slow and shallow
sweat glands	activity increased	
action within digestive tract	decreased	increased
digestive glands	decreased	increased

THE BENEFITS OF MASSAGE

1. Cell division in the epidermis is optimised resulting in an improvement in the appearance of the skin.
2. As the epidermis is being replaced frequently, the skin feels soft and smooth.
3. Skin colour is improved due to the increase in local blood circulation.
4. The collagen and elastin fibres maintain their elasticity, improving skin tone.
5. Skin texture is improved by the increased health of the epidermis and dermis.
6. Puffiness around the eyes is reduced due to the removal of excess tissue fluid.
7. Fine lines are reduced by the increased activity of the epidermis.
8. Dark circles around the eyes are reduced by the increase in blood circulation and waste removal.
9. Removal of waste products from muscle tissue prevents fatigue and gives a subsequent improvement in muscle tone.
10. Continued good lymph drainage combats the signs of ageing, resulting in the client looking young for longer.
11. Acne or spotty skins are improved as there is a reduction in the risk of infection, so fewer spots result.
12. Skin healing is improved so scarring is less likely and there may be an improvement in scars already present.
13. If spots or other infections, occur the healing process will be quicker.
14. Skin appendages benefit, in other words, hair and nails grow stronger and more quickly.

Element 6.1

Assess clients and prepare treatment plans

> **NOTE!** For further information on this element see page 103.

LOOKING AT SKIN

Accurate inspection of the skin is vital in assessing the client's needs and for the identification of contraindications. The following are contraindications specific to facial treatments. They are separated into those requiring medical referral, systemic medical conditions and those that restrict treatment within that localised area.

Contraindications requiring medical referral:
- bacterial, eg impetigo
- viral, eg herpes simplex
- fungal, eg tinea.

Contraindications that are systemic medical conditions:
- conjunctivitis

Contraindications which restrict treatment:
- recent scar tissue
- eczema
- allergies
- cuts
- abrasions
- bruising
- vitiligo
- sties.

NOTE! It is of paramount importance that you **do not** inform the client of your diagnosis of the contraindication. Instead, you should ask the client to seek medical advice from their GP. This is important as you may unduly alarm or embarrass them.

You need to understand the structure and function of the skin and the actions of the facial neck and shoulder muscles.

The key to improving the condition of the client's skin is the correct analysis.

To carry out a skin analysis you will need:
- good lighting or additional illumination
- magnifying lamp.

You must be prepared to look at the skin with care and talk to the client about their current skin care regime. Ask them to tell you about their perceptions of their skin.

NOTE! The client has come to you as a professional, an expert. Therefore, do not rely on or be mislead by the client's own diagnosis of their skin.

It is important to find out what skin type the client believes they have. This information is important, as it will provide you with clues to any anomalies you may notice during your inspection. It will also help you to make your own decision.

SKIN CHARACTERISTICS

All skin functions in basically the same way irrespective of type or colour. The colour of skin is determined by pigmentation caused by the amount of melanin present. Melanin is constantly produced to maintain the skin's natural colour. There are however important differences in the skin characteristics of people from different ethnic groups.

'White' skin

This describes those who originate from East and West Europe, North America, Canada, South Australia and New Zealand. This group are sometimes referred to as **Caucasian**. This skin has very little defence to ultra-violet light and burns easily. The group has problems with spots and blemishes, particularly through puberty but may also have a tendency towards sensitivity and dryness during their 20s and 30s. The delicate nature of the skin means that premature signs of ageing occur in the early 30s. The pale tones of the skin are usually accompanied by hair which is fair, red or mid brown.

'Yellow-toned' skin

This describes the yellowish tones of people originating from Southern Europe, South and Central America, parts of Asia, the Far East and the Middle East. This group has a tendency to skin displaying a mild oiliness, a consequence of which is a delay in the skin's ageing process. There is also more suderiferous activity. The signs of ageing will generally start during the late 30s and early 40s. This skin is prone to hyper-pigmentation and, therefore, any blemishes on this type of skin should be treated with care. Relatively minor skin damage (sometimes even expressing comedones) can lead to hyper-pigmentation. Hair colour is usually mid or dark brown to black.

'Black' skins

This describes a range of dark skins which may vary in tone from light to dark with a wide variety of undertones. There is generally more sebaceous and suderiferous activity in this group. The skin does not display signs of the ageing process until the 40s are reached. The first sign can be greying of the hair. It is easy to mistake the sheen on dark skins as excessive oiliness. The sebaceous glands are larger, however the darker the skin and more reflection of light occurs. This reflected light can be mistakenly diagnosed as too much oil. Another common mistake, particularly on dark Asian skins, is the identification of comedones on the centre 'T' panel. Close and careful examination will actually show the presence of dark facial hair around the nose and forehead not comedones. It should be noted that black skins easily form keloid scars (an over thickening of the skin) when damaged and caution should be exercised.

> **NOTE!** A lack of pigmentation, usually in irregular patches, is known as **Vitiligo**. Dark irregular patches of pigmentation is known as **Chloasma**. Corrective make-up techniques can be used to disguise both conditions.

General differences

1. Skin cancer is rare in darker skins as the pigmentation filters ultra violet radiation.
2. The epidermis on dark skins is thicker.
3. Acne is rare in darker skins despite having more sebaceous glands.
4. Paler skins are more prone to product related allergies.
5. Dark skinned people have a greater heat tolerance due to the increased number of suderiferous glands.
6. Paler skinned people have a greater tolerance to extremes of cold.
7. Black skin desquamates easily compared to white skins.

> **NOTE!** The condition of any skin will be affected by climatic changes and extremes of temperature.

SKIN TYPES

There are three main skin types you will need to identify:

1. oily
2. dry
3. combination.

Oily skin

The skin is usually coarse in texture and appears shiny, particularly around the nose, chin and forehead. You may see comedones (blackheads) and open pores, which have been stretched by a previous blockage.

The skin will appear coarse and grainy. It will appear moist and the epidermis will appear thick. It will be sallow and have a yellowish hue.

The cause of oily skin is an over secretion of sebum. It may be hormonal for example through the effects of puberty.

Dry skin

Dry skin appears taut and tight, fine lines may be evident and there may be flaky patches. There is a tendency for dilated capillaries; these are the permanent dilation of tiny capillary blood vessels. Blood has leaked from the capillaries leaving a spidery appearance across the cheekbones and around the nose.

The skin will be fine in texture, sensitive and finely lined but will have a coarse surface. It would be unlikely that the skin would have any comedones or open pores.

The causes of dry skin are:

- not enough sebum, with low fluid content in the upper layers of the skin
- excessive use of soaps and degreasing agents such as astringents
- exposure to sunlight without due care and attention
- extremes of temperature
- central heating will also have a drying effect.

Combination skin

The face has a central panel commonly referred to as the 'T' zone, which includes the forehead, nose and chin. In this skin type these areas will appear oily and congested, whilst the rest of the skin may be dry. This is one of the most common skin types.

SKIN CONDITIONS

You will also need to recognise and differentiate between skin types and skin conditions. The following are skin conditions that you should be able to identify:

- sensitive
- dehydrated
- mature
- seborrhoea
- milia
- comedone.

Sensitive skin

Sensitive skin is thin; it blotches easily and is quickly irritated. It may be recognised by its high colour and warmth. There may be fine dilated capillaries around the cheeks and nose.

Dehydrated skin

Dehydrated skin lacks moisture and appears dull. It may become itchy and tight. It may also have a smooth sheen but you must not confuse this characteristic with that of oily skin. Any skin type can become dehydrated and it is considered a temporary condition.

Mature skin

This condition describes skin that has started the ageing process. It lacks oil and moisture. Character lines and wrinkles are beginning to form around the muscles of facial expression. There is some loss of underlying muscle tone and the subcutaneous (fatty) layer is shrinking.

Seborrhoea

Seborrhoeic conditions are caused by over-active sebaceous glands, creating too much sebum on a skin, which is already naturally oily.

It is a common condition in young people and is particularly associated with the onset of puberty. It may also cause acne if it is left untreated. The sebaceous secretions are increased and the skin becomes grainy with enlarged pores and comedones. The pores can become blocked with the sebaceous secretions. As the hormones settle down, the condition subsides.

Milia

Milia is the name given to sebum trapped within a blind duct. It is common on dry skin types, particularly around the eye and cheek area. It appears as a white pearly nodule and is a clear indication of a tendency towards dryness in that localised area. If the milia is not established it may be possible to disperse with gentle massage. If however it is a hardened mass then it will be necessary to remove it using a sterile lance on prewarmed skin. The top of the milia is split using the sterile lance and the milia is lifted out. The skin is then left to heal. Milia should never be expressed in the way that comedones may be. It would cause the client a great deal of discomfort and may lead to permanent damage of the skin.

Comedone

A comedone is the term given to a blackhead. Comedones are formed when sebum is trapped within a pore; keratinised cells at the top of the pore multiply and block off the exit from the sebaceous gland. The surface of the blocked pore becomes black due to oxidation (a chemical reaction when exposed to air). When there is a build up of sebum it may cause the gland to erupt, which will allow sebum into the lower levels of the skin. When this occurs it leads into the formulation of a papule. If it becomes infected it will become a pustule.

THE DANGER TRIANGLE

The danger triangle covers an area from the centre of the eyebrows at its tip spreading outwards to the lower lip at its base. The client should be advised not to express spots around this area. There are important blood vessels, which lie directly under the triangle, and if the skin is damaged they may be prone to bacterial infection. This may cause a condition known as **deep cavernous thrombosis**.

AGEING AND THE SKIN

The general characteristics of ageing usually occur around the age of 40 or with the onset of the menopause. Skin ages at different rates depending upon several factors. These may include ethnic group, hereditary or health-related factors and the treatment it has received. Incorrect cleansing, harsh treatment, overexposure to ultraviolet light, smoking and extremes of temperature all play a part in the ageing process. Despite the best possible skin care regime the underlying muscle structure tends to lose its tone and inevitably a softening of the features occurs.

The softening of the skin and decrease in muscle tone creates character lines, particularly around the muscles of expression. There is a loss of elasticity in the skin and the expression lines become permanent. This effect is caused by the break down of collagen and elastin fibres within the dermis. It is the bundles of collagen which make the young skin supple and smooth.

The formation of wrinkles occurs along the lines of facial expression. This is why wrinkles are often referred to as character lines! The regular contraction of the muscle forms the lines and, whilst the skin can stretch easily, it cannot contract in the same way as muscles. Thus as the skin loses its elasticity the lines become more and more etched.

A combination of these factors clearly indicates the onset of the ageing process. The appearance of the skin reflects the underlying changes.

The physical and physiological signs of ageing

The following features are signs of ageing skin:

1. Circulation slows down therefore waste is not removed as efficiently.
2. The elasticity of the skin decreases and character lines are formed.
3. There is an accelerated growth of fine lanugo or baby hair particularly on the cheek and upper lip.
4. There is a decrease of skin permeability leading to gradual dehydration.
5. There is an increase in hyper pigmentation for example chloasma (liver spots).
6. The skin becomes noticeably thinner especially around the eyes.
7. The capillary network can be more easily ruptured due to the inelasticity of the skin.
8. There is a decrease in sebum production.
9. There is a decrease in the activity of the suderiferous glands.
10. The basal cell metabolic rate slows down.
11. There are open pores present.

ANALYSING SKIN

The skin will tell you a story: you will be able to look at a client with a mature skin condition and immediately identify the type of skin that they had in earlier life. It will tell you if the client was predisposed to be a particular skin type.

> **NOTE!** An open pore is an empty one! At some stage, it has been enlarged through a blockage, excess oil or a blemish in that area.

You must be careful not to make a superficial diagnosis. A common error is to examine the skin, but fail to talk to the client about their skin care routine and their own perceptions of their skin. Correct analysis is like an investigation, which will require good detective work to find the clues and piece them together. It is important to gather as much information as possible. The client may be using inappropriate products, which are stripping the skin's protective acid mantle. This leaves the skin feeling taut, shiny, prone to infection and bacterial invasion. Clients may feel that their skin is oily because of the effect of using these products and will mistakenly use a product for oily skin, which will be too harsh and will exacerbate the problem.

> **NOTE!** The more the client uses inappropriate products, the more the body attempts to restore the acid mantle through increased secretions. This may lead to even more shine!

The group who are most likely to fall into this trap are those going through puberty. Companies still tend to target this vulnerable group with products so harsh they can upset the delicate skin balance at an early age. Incorrect selection of products can also sensitise areas. If the product is too strong, it can induce vascular response which can result in the underlying capillaries stretching or dilating. In some cases the capillaries may rupture.

Look out for clients who use sunbeds or those who have recently been exposed to sunlight. They will display signs of dehydrated skin but remember this is likely to be a temporary state. A note should be made on the record card and subsequent changes recorded. The range of false or self-tanning products, whilst harmless, can affect an effective diagnosis. It is possible, weeks after application, when the skin colour has normalised to have open pores still stained with the product. The clear liquid type products are more likely to do this than the cream formulations. It may require a series of exfoliating treatments to remove the problem. Clients should be advised of the correct application of such products.

> **NOTE!** The therapist must take care when analysing darker skins, as imperfections readily visible on a lighter skin may not be immediately noticeable.

It is important not to rush the skin analysis and you should allow at least 5 minutes for a thorough analysis in the treatment schedule.

> **NOTE!** It is important that you treat the current condition of the skin. It is of vital importance that you conduct a thorough analysis each time the client visits and you must note all changes.

Establishing the correct skin category, in terms of skin type and condition, has implications for the effectiveness of the recommended treatment.

The systems for recording findings will differ from one salon to another. It is usual for salons to design their own system of record cards based on their 'house' style. Salons also use treatment plans. A treatment plan is a record of the proposed schedule of treatment and the therapist's recommendations. Plans may be one double sided form or may be two separate ones (see page 108).

Remember a treatment plan should include:
- Client's full name
- Client's usual skin care routine
- Result of skin analysis

- Recommended treatments and products – including costs and duration
- Outcomes of treatment
- Contraindications
- Contra-actions
- Aftercare advice given
- Client's signature
- Record of client feedback

A record card should include:

- Client's full name
- Client's address and telephone number(s)
- Date of birth
- Doctor's address and telephone number
- Medical history

It is important to record your findings neatly; other therapists may need to refer to the records.

Activity

1 Design a treatment plan and record card that encompasses all of the listed characteristics in the 'house' style that best suits your salon environment (an example can be found on page 108).

2 List five important questions to ask your client during an initial consultation.

SELLING IN THE SALON

Beauty therapy trainees have always found selling within the salon environment a difficult concept to grasp! They are usually very able when it comes to putting together a suitable treatment plan but for some reason find selling products very difficult. If you can sell a service (a treatment) then logically you should be able to sell a product. More emphasis is now placed on retailing in training situations and you will be expected to retail alongside the recommended treatment. Retailing is now part of the therapist's role and is a very important one. It benefits the clients in that they are purchasing products from a professional range that the therapist has recommended. Beauty therapists usually receive commission on products sold, so this is a good way of increasing your salary!

NOTE! Link selling is a good opportunity to promote new colours and products, for example, a lipcolour with a matching nail enamel.

The advice you have given to the client about the products you have used and the recommended aftercare must be clearly recorded on the record card or treatment plan. This should be discussed within the privacy of the treatment room so that the client is clear about the items required at the reception or sales area (see page 110).

Find the gap in the client's product range and fill it rather than insisting she purchase all the products. If the product is more appropriate for her, she will purchase more.

Stock

It is important that you know your way around the stockroom! The shelving should be adjustable and easy to clean. Shelving should be labelled and popular lines should be stored at eye level.

It is important to keep a note of how particular products are selling and then to inform the Salon Supervisor, Manager or whoever has responsibility for ordering stock.

Displays

The reception area is one of the most important areas in the salon. It is here that the client will be greeted and here that the client will sit either before or after treatment. Vital then that the best opportunity is made of this area. There should be attractive displays that highlight treatments and product range. The displays should be changed every few weeks to maintain client interest and to demonstrate that the salon is keeping abreast of new treatments and products. A well thought out display area will attract clients and will increase salon profitability.

> **NOTE!** Tips for displays:
> - keep them dust free
> - have a theme
> - reflect the season ie Christmas
> - have testers/samples available
> - restock often
> - do not have gaps!

PRODUCTS

You must be familiar with the range of available products in order to make the correct selection for each individual client. You need to know which products are required for each treatment.

Cleansers

A good cleansing medium should:
- remove make-up, dirt and grime effectively
- be suitable for the client's needs
- be easily applied and easily removed.

There are several types of cleansing preparation available: creams, milks, lotions, soapless cleansers and bars.

Creams

These are ideal for mature skin conditions and for dry skin types. They are designed to dissolve the pigmented waxes that are found in make-up products. They are usually water in oil emulsions and therefore do not soak into the skin. They have a cooling effect on the skin and are easily removed.

Milks

These are available in various consistencies. Most milks are emulsions and are made from oil in a water solution. They are not very effective in removing a heavy make-up and are mainly used for superficial cleansing.

Lotions

Cleansing lotions are particularly useful on congested or oily skin. They leave very little residual oil on the skin after removal. However, they can be very strong so it is important that you know the product and that the skin has been accurately analysed.

Soapless cleansers and cleansing bars

These products are becoming the popular choice. They have changed the concept of cleansing, particularly in relation to the male market. Many clients will inform you that they prefer to use soap and water because they do not feel that their skin has been properly cleansed otherwise. This range of products now allows clients to use a more gentle complexion soap with water. Cleansing bars are made from soft soap but have a carefully balanced pH, which does not leave the skin feeling tight and shiny. They leave the skin at the correct pH balance and are particularly effective on seborrhoeic and acne skins. Soapless cleansers are made from laurel sulphates and soap bars contain potassium palmitate.

Toners

Toner is used at the conclusion of the cleansing treatment and prepares the skin for make-up application. It removes any product remaining on the skin after cleansing or facemask removal. Toners dissolve surface oil and have an anti-bacterial effect. They may also have a refreshing effect depending upon the type selected. Toner refines the pore size as it evaporates, leaving the skin prepared for an application of moisturiser.

Toners are made from infusions of herbs and flowers, such as witch hazel, orange flower water, rose water, and small amounts of glycerine in distilled water. Other ingredients could include zinc sulphate and potassium sulphate. Toners also contain varying amounts of alcohol, which determines their strength.

As with cleansing products, there are a wide range to choose from.

Skin tonics
This range includes astringent solutions, which can be very strong. The amount of alcohol present and the active ingredient, for example witch hazel, will determine which tonic you select for a particular client's skin. If more than 20 per cent alcohol is present use should be restricted to oily skin types. An astringent removes the surface oil and can disturb the skin pH balance. It would therefore be contraindicated on blemished or sensitive conditions as it could be an irritant. Witch hazel has astringent properties and also should be used with caution.

Skin fresheners and bracers
These have a much gentler effect. The action is a refreshing but mild one and these products are suitable for dehydrated, dry, delicate and mature skin conditions. They contain only small amounts of alcohol and do not remove oil as efficiently as their stronger counterparts. A dilution of orange flower water or rose water is an example.

Eye make-up cleansers
These specially designed products need to have certain characteristics. They must not be heavy in texture, highly perfumed or excessively creamy, but must be effective in removing densely pigmented waterproof products. They are based on a mineral oil such as liquid paraffin or soft waxes such as paraffin wax.

Activity
1 What are the main differences between a skin tonic and a skin freshener?
2 What are the qualities required of an eye make-up remover?
3 What is the acid mantle?

Exfoliants
Exfoliants aid desquamation (the skin's natural shedding of surface cells). They smooth the surface of the skin, prepare the skin for further treatment, and stimulate the blood and lymphatic flow thereby aiding the elimination and absorption of waste products. All skin types benefit from using exfoliating products.

They fall into two categories: pore grains or facial scrubs and peeling creams.

Pore grains or facial scrubs
These are made from grains of detergent and small pieces of almond meal, oatmeal, and pumice or ground fruit kernels. They have a detergent cleansing action and when gently massaged over

the skin remove surface adhesions, leaving the skin soft and smooth. Their regular use should be restricted to those with an oily skin and only limited usage for those wishing to refine and tone.

Peeling creams

These are based on clay and other natural biological ingredients. They are applied to the skin and allowed to dry. They can then be lifted off the skin or gently rolled using friction to slough off dead cells. These are effective on all skin types particularly those conditions which require gentle treatment.

Exfoliation treatments

Brush cleanse is an intensive cleansing treatment. It has an exfoliating effect by loosening surface adhesions and increases blood circulation creating warmth. It can also be used to remove specialised exfoliating facemasks. The machine comprises of a series of brushes which, when attached to the motor driven applicator, rotate at varying speeds dependant upon need and purpose. There is a variety of brush heads available:

- soft complexion brushes – these are used for general cleansing purposes
- sponge heads – these are usually used with a foaming cleansing product and are a gentler alternative to the brushes
- bristle brush heads – these are used for a more stimulating effect and are good for working on male clients
- pumice block – this is used for peeling and refining a coarse skin texture.

Preparation of the skin

The skin should be cleansed to remove make-up and surface oil. A suitable medium should then be applied. The choice of medium will depend on need. You can choose from a variety of liquid detergent based cleansing products to cleansing creams.

Safety precautions

- It is important to ensure that a uniform pressure is applied.
- Do not over wet the brush head as you will spray the cleansing product everywhere!
- Use a dampened cotton wool pad or sponge to protect the eyes and mouth.
- Choose the brush head and medium with care.
- Avoid dragging the skin.
- Avoid over stimulation of the skin.
- Ensure the brush heads are clean and sterilised before and after use.

Contraindications

This treatment would be contraindicated for those with a sensitive skin condition or loose crepey skin.

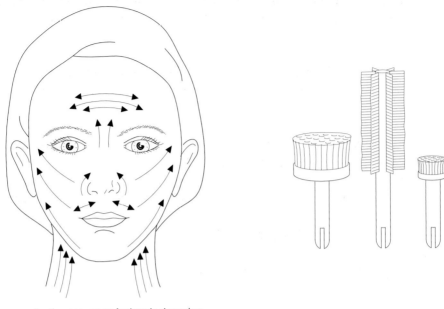

application sequence for brush cleansing

Figure 6.14 A brush cleanse treatment

Activity

1 What is exfoliation?

2 State two precautions to take when using exfoliants.

Massage mediums

Massage can be carried out using a variety of mediums. Most however will be based on either a cream or an oil formulation, which may have added ingredients to suit the individual needs of the client's skin. Mediums contain mineral oils, beeswax or paraffin wax and a large percentage of distilled water.

Moisturisers

Moisturisers comprise of an oil and water emulsion. They can be presented in either a cream or liquid form.

They readily evaporate from the skin leaving a fine film of **emollient**. An emollient is a substance which softens the skin by increasing its water content and keeps it soft by slowing moisture loss. The gentle evaporation produces a cooling sensation, which temporarily refines the pores and leaves the skin feeling soft and supple. The moisturiser leaves an aqueous film on the skin which is ready for make-up to be applied.

Moisturisers also supplement the skin's water content by the attraction of water from the atmosphere by the means of a **humectant** (water attracting) product. Humectant materials are glycerol, sorbitol and glycol.

All skin types require the use of a moisturiser. Moisturisers prolong the appearance of make-up; they prepare the skin for the application of foundation by smoothing the surface. They also protect the skin from the pigments in the make-up. Moisturiser should always be worn even if make-up is not; it will protect the skin from the elements and pollutants in the atmosphere.

The choice of moisturiser will depend on skin type.

> **NOTE!** Always check the content of products, particularly toners. Manufacturers are now legally required to list product ingredients.

SPECIALIST SKIN PRODUCTS

Eye creams, gels and lotions

These specialist products are used to temporarily minimise the appearance of crows feet and character lines; they may also have a temporary tightening effect. The creams are formulated in the same way as moisturisers. They contain cocoa butter and vegetable oils. Petroleum jelly and high wax content are avoided as they can cause puffiness around the delicate eye area. Eye gels often contain astringents such as witch hazel. They have a cooling and firming effect on the delicate tissue surrounding the eyes. Lotions are similar to gels. They are usually applied onto a dampened pad of cotton wool and placed over the eyes. They produce a soothing, refreshing effect on the eyes.

Acne products

There are certain products, which are now recognised as irritants to acne. These are products which contain petroleum jelly, lanolin and some vegetable oils. There are specifically designed lotions, which are spirit-based in a chemical formulation to prevent infections. The use of soapless cleansers and complexion soaps as described earlier in this unit are particularly effective on acnefied skins.

Neck creams

Neck creams are rich moisturising creams that may contain other active ingredients such as collagen. The action of these rich formulations is primarily to soften, tighten and tone the skin.

Lip balms

These are a range of specifically designed products for softening and protecting the lips. They form a protective film and prevent moisture loss. They are formulated from varying mixtures of oils and waxes and may contain colour pigments or are presented in their natural state.

Night creams

Night creams are emollients and they are generally heavier and thicker than other skin creams. They are usually formulated from a range of products including animal fats, vegetable oils, cocoa butter, olive and almond oils and beeswax. The action of a night cream is to soften and hydrate the skin. Most products contain a humectant.

Activity

1 State three reasons why using a moisturiser is important.

2 List two qualities of an eye gel, cream or lotion.

Element 6.2

Prepare the client and work area for treatment

PREPARATION FOR TREATMENT

Reception

The visual appearance of the salon and the manner in which the client is greeted is of vital importance. It is essential that there is a professional atmosphere at all times, in which the client feels comfortable and uninhibited. If the atmosphere at the reception is professional, it will instil confidence in the client.

NOTE! Every person who walks through the door is a potential client for not only one, but many of the salon services. Know your services and products!

Personal appearance

The client is coming to you for a range of treatments and services that will help to maintain or improve a particular condition or meet a specific need. You are therefore perceived to be a professional, an exponent of your craft. It is important that your image projects your expertise! Your appearance will indicate to others how much care and pride you take in your role. Clients will judge you on your image and the beauty business is one in which the correct image and appearance are paramount. You may be very confident and knowledgeable in the services and products offered, but if your image is not appropriate it sends the wrong message to the client. See Unit 1 which deals with personal appearance in more detail.

> **NOTE!** You only have one chance to make a first impression!

PREPARATION OF TREATMENT AREA

Safe and hygienic practices within a salon environment are crucial to prevent cross infection. Tools, materials and equipment must be sterilised before and after each client. Linen should also be changed after each client. The recognition of contraindications is of vital importance to prevent cross infection.

It is essential to create a calm and relaxing environment for the client. The salon furnishings and equipment should be appropriate and fit for the purpose.

It is likely that the client will be apprehensive, particularly if it is their first visit. It is important to avoid delays and you should have everything prepared and ready for the clients arrival. It will also increase salon efficiency if you work within the time parameters for each treatment. You should check your column in the appointment book before commencing work and refer to salon records of previous visits where appropriate. If it is a new client, you should have all necessary paperwork ready for completion. You should also check the range of products available to ensure you can offer a range of options to suit the individual need and recommendations following initial consultation.

Trolley
Remember, visual impressions count! The trolley should be clean and tidy and contain all the products needed to carry out the required service or treatment.

You should have on your trolley:
- cotton wool – dry and dampened – to remove cleansing products and for applying products such as toners
- tissues – to blot the skin and to remove cleansing products
- a selection of bowls – for holding dry cotton wool, for holding dampened cotton wool
- spatulas – to remove creams and products from containers, to mix face mask formulation
- a selection of skin care products – always remember to replace lids, use spatulas to remove products or in the case of liquid products pour into the palm of your hand

- face mask brush – to apply formulation (do not remove from steriliser until ready to be used)
- facial sponges – to remove product, to remove face mask formulation
- a covered waste receptacle.

You should also have ready and prepared:
- record card or treatment plan
- protective headband
- towels
- hand mirror.

Facials are performed on the client in a reclining or semi-reclining position. The treatment chair or couch should be capable of adapting to meet the requirements of the treatment. The height of the couch is important both for client comfort and for the beauty therapist. Back problems are common amongst therapists and, therefore, it is important to prevent such problems by correct positioning. The beauty therapist normally works from behind the client and may be seated or may stand to carry out the treatment. There should be pillows and covering available for the client during treatment to provide warmth and to promote relaxation. If you are working in a cubicle, it should have screening, which will ensure complete privacy from the rest of the salon.

You should have a steamer and brush cleanse unit available.

The client

The client should be given very clear instructions about what to do. Hair and clothing should be protected. You should ask the client to remove their outer clothing and you should offer them a robe or towel to protect their modesty. It would be expected that privacy would be a paramount consideration. You should ask the client to remove all necklaces and earrings.

Once the client is settled on the chair or couch ask them to remove or slip down any straps which will inhibit the facial treatment.

The client's head should be slightly elevated and their hair should be protected using a headband or other suitable covering. Finally, wash your hands – you are now ready to commence treatment.

> **NOTE!** Always ensure that your client sees you wash your hands. This will instil confidence and demonstrate good hygienic practice.

Activity

1 Describe how you think a beauty therapist should present themselves. Discuss your findings with a colleague.

2 State what should be on the trolley for a facial.

Element 6.3

Improve skin condition using skin care and massage techniques

THE FACIAL

Cleansing

Cleansing usually comprises of two stages. The first stage is to superficially remove surface oil and make-up. The second stage is to thoroughly deep cleanse the skin. The analysis of the skin type will be carried out after the superficial cleanse. You may be expected to conduct cleansing in a routine that has been adopted as the 'house style' in your salon or training institute. Inevitably, the routine will be based upon common principles and practices.

> **NOTE!** Always check for contraindications.

Procedure for a superficial cleanse

This is always carried out, whether the client is wearing make-up or not.

1. Ask the client to close their eyes and select a suitable cleansing product.
2. Apply the selected product using small gentle circular movements. Avoid exerting too much pressure over the eye. Apply to upper lid, lashes and under the eye.
3. If the client is wearing mascara, place a dampened pad of cotton wool under the lashes and apply eye make-up remover with either fingers or cotton bud until the mascara has dissolved.
4. Remove the loosened make-up and cleanser using dampened cotton wool pads. Ensure you support the skin as you work.
5. Select a suitable product for the lip area. Apply using gentle circular movements.
6. Remove the loosened lip cosmetic and cleanser with dampened cotton wool. Blot the lips using a tissue.
7. Select a suitable product for the face and neck. Apply the selected product using light upward movements on the cheeks, forehead and neck. Work the product into the folds around the nose and chin.
8. Remove the cleanser product by initially blotting with soft facial tissues. Tissues are used for their absorbency when using greasy or oil based products. Dampened cotton

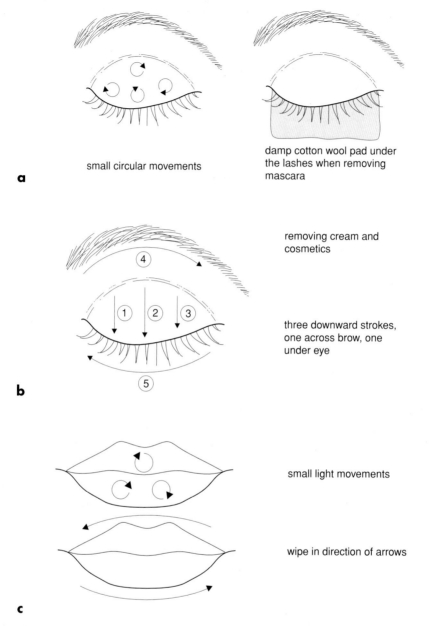

small circular movements

damp cotton wool pad under the lashes when removing mascara

a

removing cream and cosmetics

three downward strokes, one across brow, one under eye

b

small light movements

wipe in direction of arrows

c

Figure 6.15 a b c Steps in a superficial cleanse

wool may be used to remove water-soluble debris from the skin. The skin is clean when the cotton wool shows no soiling.

9. Apply a light application of mild toner using dampened cotton wool pads.
10. Blot the skin using a facial tissue. Place a hole in the centre for the nose and blot. Then fold the tissue down onto the neck and blot again.

11. You should allow at least 5 minutes in the treatment schedule for superficial cleansing.

> **NOTE!** Always cleanse the lip and eye areas first. This will ensure these areas are thoroughly cleansed and will prevent the spreading of densely pigmented make-up over the face and neck.

Deep cleanse

The analysis of the skin should take place before commencing the deep cleanse. Analysis should be carried out at each visit and you should not simply accept the previous diagnosis (see page 159).

The aim of the deep cleanse is to:
- soften and loosen comedones and other skin blockages
- increase circulation
- remove any remaining make-up preparation
- increase desquamation.

It is important that you adapt movements and pressure according to client need. Each movement should be repeated at least six times unless otherwise stated.

Procedure for a deep cleanse

Select a suitable cleansing product.

1. Place hands at the base of the neck. Work upwards over the platysma muscle to the jaw (mandible bone), using a light flowing movement. Sweep across the mandible. Apply a light sweeping stroke down either side of the neck following the sterno-mastoid muscles.
2. Using a light sweeping movement work along the mandible from one side to the other.
3. Starting at the chin use small circular movements moving slowly up to the sides of the nose. Glide along the cheeks (zygomatic muscle and zygomatic bone) without exerting pressure and back to the chin.
4. Slide hands along each cheekbone and up to the forehead. Gently slide the hands down over the nose and back along the cheek.
5. Using small circular movements work around the base of the nose.
6. Slide the fingers down the top and sides of the nose using alternating strokes.
7. Using large circular movements work across the forehead, slide across the cheekbone and back up to the forehead.
8. Using the pads of the fingers perform a scissor or zigzag movement across the fore-head working from one side to the other.
9. Stroke around each eye using ring finger and gently perform a lifting movement, three times under each eyebrow.
   Always conclude a facial routine by applying slight pressure at the temples, which indicates the end of routine.
   Remove cleansing product by blotting the surface with tissues then using dampened cotton wool pads. It is vitally important to ensure all trace of cleanser is removed. You

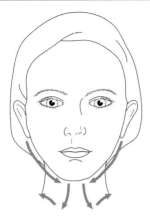

1

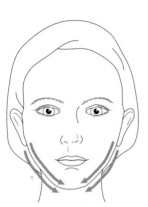

2

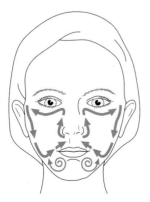

3

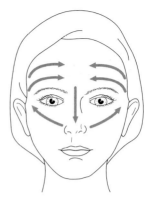

4

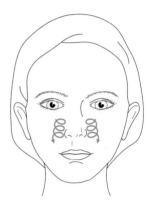

5

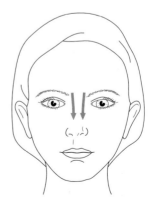

6

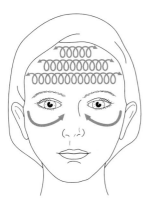

7

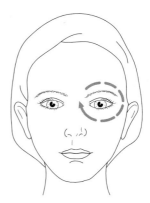

9

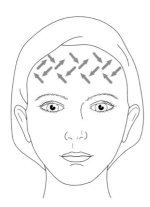

8

Figure 6.16 1 to 9 Steps in a deep cleanse

should check around the hairline, under the jaw and in the folds of the skin. You may then apply toner.

You should allow at least 10 minutes for deep cleansing in the treatment schedule.

> **NOTE!** Always work the chosen cleansing medium between both hands to warm the product and to provide slip.

Extractions
Comedones

Comedones will have been loosened following a deep cleanse and extraction of skin blockages can take place at this point. The skin should be warmed using either hot dampened cotton wool pads or by using a steamer.

Steaming

The steamer should be filled in accordance with manufacturer's instructions. It is usual to fill the steamer using distilled water. This prevents the element furring up with limescale, which can cause the unit to spit boiling water.

The duration of treatment will vary between 3 and 20 minutes. Positioning of the unit will depend upon skin type:

- 25 cm (10 in) for an oily skin
- 30 cm (12 in) for normal skin
- 40 cm (15 in) for a dry skin.

If the client has dilated capillaries or has very sensitive skin you should avoid stimulating the circulation and, therefore, steaming would not be indicated.

Most steamers have an ozone facility within the unit. The use of ozone is particularly beneficial to those who have a blemished skin. It is drying and has an anti-bacterial effect. There are restrictions governing the use of ozone, however, and it is important that you check with your local health authority before offering the facility. The ozone option is not required for warming the skin.

You must make all the precautionary safety checks before using a steaming unit:

- Ensure that the unit is not over filled.
- Make sure that it is on a safe, solid base.
- Place the unit at the correct distance for the skin type.
- There should be no trailing wires or flexes.
- Check that the vapour is evenly emitted before directing toward the client.

When steaming has been completed, the skin should be blotted. Extractions should be carried out using fingers covered with tissue or a comedone extractor. If the fingers are used, a rolling pressing motion should be used until the comedone is expressed. If a comedone remover is used then gentle even pressure should be applied over the blockage. You should work with caution to prevent exerting too much pressure which may cause bruising.

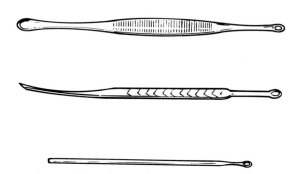

Figure 6.17 Types of comedome extractor

Milia

Milia should also be removed following steaming. They however should never be expressed by exerting pressure. They are usually formed into a hard pearly lump when they have become established. Following steaming the milia is gently exposed and using a sterile lance the lump is lifted out. Great care must be taken to prevent infection.

Activity

1 State the differences between a superficial cleanse and a deep cleanse.

2 What precautions should be taken when carrying out extractions?

FACIAL MASSAGE

All good facial treatments should be aimed at improving the skin tone and texture, firming the underlying muscles and tissue structure. A good facial massage will cleanse, tone and refine the skin, strengthen the muscles and relax the client. The stimulation of the circulation will increase cell regeneration and will maintain the correct oil and fluid balance of the skin. By understanding the classification of massage movements and their effects, the therapist can tailor a massage to suit the need of the individual client.

The facial massage is based around four types of movements – **effleurage**, **petrissage**, **tapotement** and **vibrations**. Each of these movements has a specific purpose. You may be expected to learn a routine that has been designed as the salon or training institute's 'house style'. Whatever routine is adopted, it will be based on these four massage movements.

Effleurage

Massage always starts with effleurage. This is a series of light, continuous stroking movements that are designed to relax the client and are used to link up other movements and manipulations within the routine.

Effects of effleurage:
- increases blood circulation
- increases lymphatic drainage
- aids desquamation
- promotes relaxation.

Petrissage

Petrissage is a series of compression movements, which include kneading, knuckling, lifting, rolling and pinching. The movements are intermittent and deeper than those employed in effleurage. They are used over soft tissue.

Effects of petrissage:
- increases the blood circulation
- improves lymphatic drainage
- improves muscle tone
- increases mitosis
- aids desquamation.

Tapotement

Tapotement movements are applied in a light, quick, stimulating manner. They include movements such as slapping and tapping. They should be applied in a continuous rhythmic series of strokes.

Effects of tapotement:
- stimulates the nerve endings
- increases blood circulation
- improves lymphatic drainage
- tones the skin.

Vibration

Vibrations are applied by producing a quick contraction and relaxation of the therapist's arm muscles. The client experiences a light trembling sensation.

Effects of vibrations:
- relaxing
- stimulates the nerve endings

The overall effects of facial massage are:
- increases blood and lymphatic circulation
- increases mitosis (the process by which cells reproduce)
- improves skin texture
- promotes relaxation.

The repetition of movements will depend upon the needs of the individual client. The routine should take between 15 and 20 minutes. The selection of a suitable massage medium will depend upon client need, but will usually be a cream or oil-based product.

Procedure for a facial massage

1. Place fingers on the pectoral muscle at the base of the sternum. Slide across and around the shoulder (deltoid muscle). Turn the hands and slide back along the trapezius muscle to the neck.
2. Slide the fingers to the deltoid and use circular thumb kneading along the trapezius to the top of the spine. Slide back and repeat.
3. Place the fingers on trapezius, at deltoid, and proceed with deep circular finger kneading.

4. Place the fingers at the back of the neck and vibrate up the back of the neck.
5. Circular kneading along platysma and sterno-mastoid.
6. Cup hands one above the other, place on the sternum, slide up the left side of the neck, across the jawline and down the right side.
7. Bend the fingers and using the knuckles, knuckle up and down the neck area.
8. Place the thumbs on the centre of the chin. With first fingers placed under the jaw, slide the thumbs firmly down the platysma, bring the first fingers onto the chin, slide along the jawline to the ear, change and slide down to the chin.
9. Place the thumbs one above the other on the chin and proceed with circular kneading along the jawline to the ear and back. Reverse the circling and knead to the other ear.
10. Place the thumbs at the corners of the mouth and lift the mouth with a flicking upward movement.
11. Clasp the fingers under the chin, turn hands, unclasp and slide the hands up the face towards the forehead.
12. Place the hands on the forehead at the temples and stroke upwards from the eyebrow to the hairline from left to right.
13. Using the ring finger draw a figure of eight around the eyes.
14. Repeat movement 11.
15. Circular kneading from the chin to the nose to the temples.
16. With thumbs on the cheeks, carry out deep circular kneading to the cheek area.
17. From left to right, tap along the jawline.
18. Cup the hands and lift the masseter muscle on each side of the face and release.
19. Using thumb and forefinger, proceed with a deep rolling pinching movement to the cheek area.
20. Place the pads of the fingers on the mandible and proceed to work towards the ear, using a lifting movement.
21. Knuckle along the jawline and on the cheek area.
22. Using the palm of the hand slap along the jawline from ear to ear lifting the muscles.
23. Repeat movement.
24. Scissor movement to forehead.
25. Using pads of the fingers tap gently around the eye area.
26. Repeat movement 13.
27. Repeat movement 1.
28. Slide the hands across to the temples and apply slight pressure to signify the end of the routine.

Activity

1   What adaptations could you make to the facial massage routine for a client with dry or sensitive skin?

2   How much time should you allow for the facial massage?

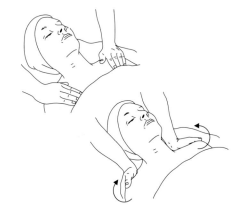

1

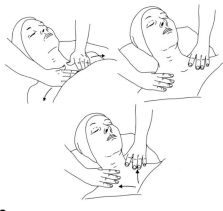

2

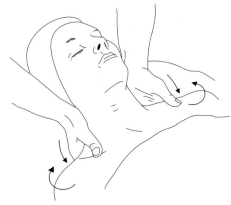

3

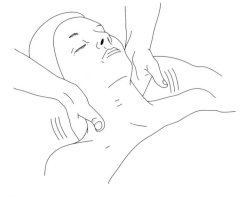

4

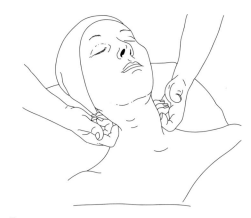

5

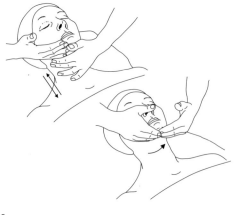

6

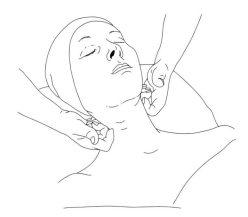

7

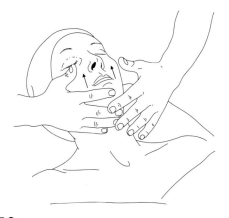

10

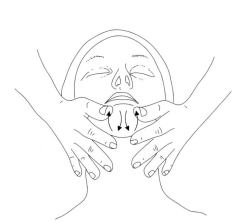

8

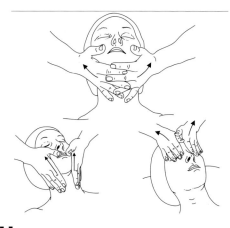

11

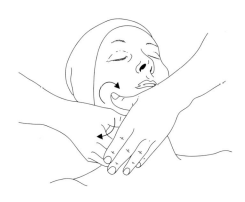

9

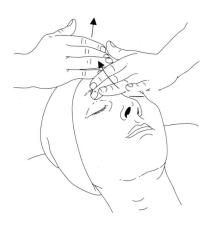

12

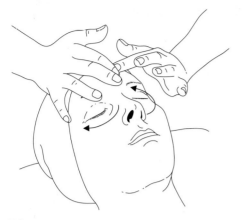

13

14 Repeat movement 11

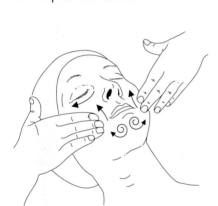

15

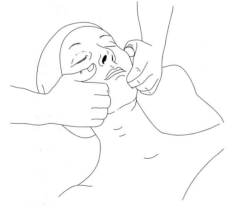

16

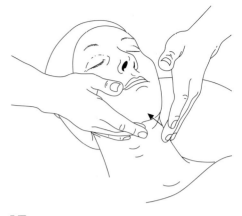

17

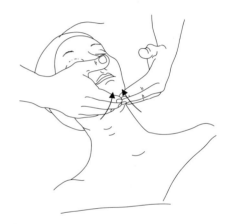

18

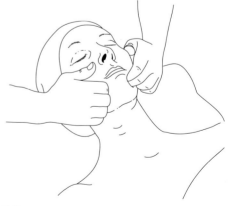

19

23 Repeat movement 11

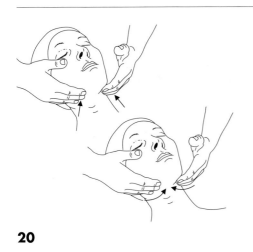

20

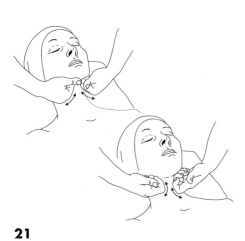

21

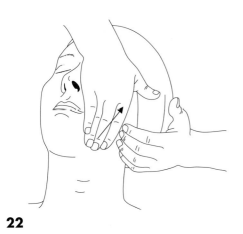

22

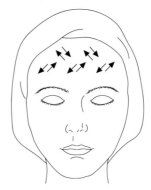

24

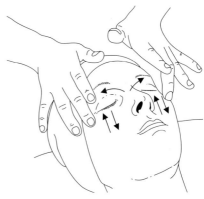

25

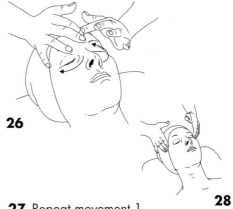

26

28

27 Repeat movement 1

Figure 6.18 1 to 28 Steps in a facial massage

FACE MASKS

Face masks complement the beneficial effects of the cleansing routine. They have deep cleansing qualities and may contain active ingredients.

Face masks are based upon different formulations which will vary according to the ingredients used and the action required. A sound knowledge of the action and effects of the basic ingredients will allow you to formulate preparations to suit the need of the individual. The timings for face masks within the treatment schedule will vary depending on the type selected, however a face mask doesn't usually take more than 20 minutes.

The mask is generally applied at the end of the facial treatment. However some facial routines may specify the application of the mask at a specific point designed to achieve maximum benefit.

There are several types of mask used to suit all skin types:
- **Setting masks** – these masks dry on the skin. They include clay-based masks and peel off masks.
- **Non-setting masks** – these masks do not set but are cooling and soothing on the skin. They include biological and clay-based masks, to which oil is added.
- **Specialised masks** – these are masks which include paraffin wax, oil masks, gel masks, thermal masks and cream masks.

Face masks have many beneficial effects on the skin. They:
- soothe and calm
- soften
- improve desquamation
- moisturise
- deep cleanse
- slight bleaching effect
- remove excess oil
- stimulate circulation.

General contraindications to face masks are as follows:
- infections like herpes simplex or impetigo
- recent scar tissue
- cuts and abrasions
- highly sensitive or sensitised skin, for example through sunburn

The mask should be applied onto skin which has been thoroughly cleansed and is free of all products. In some cases the mask may be applied over the massage medium when carrying out specialised treatments. However, normally the skin will be completely free of all traces of product. Earlier in this unit skin analysis and inspection was discussed (see page 159). It is very important that you examine the skin thoroughly to enable you to make an informed decision about the most suitable formulation for the client.

The mask should be mixed with a spatula, not a brush. This will ensure an even distribution of ingredients. If a brush is used to mix, the neck of the brush becomes clogged with the formula. Masks can be applied with a brush or spatula depending on type. They should be applied evenly, especially clay-based masks mixed to a setting formula. If they are unevenly applied they can evaporate too quickly giving a burning, itching sensation on the skin.

Soothing, refreshing eye pads made from witch hazel or water can be applied. Client preference however should be ascertained as some clients may feel claustrophobic and prefer to have their eyes open.

Setting masks
Clay-based masks

Clay masks are made from a variety of clay and powdered mineral ingredients. The basic ingredients are:

- **Calamine** – this is a pale pink powder. It is ideal for sensitive skin conditions. It soothes inflamed skin, calms high colour and has a very gentle effect. It is usually mixed with orange flower water or rose water.
- **Magnesium carbonate** – this is a bright white powder. It has slightly astringent properties and is particularly effective on skins with isolated blemishes. It is commonly used in conjunction with other powders because of its effects.
- **Kaolin** – this is a dull white powder, stronger in effect than magnesium carbonate. It has a drawing effect which is deep cleansing. It increases blood circulation and removal of waste products.
- **Fullers earth** – this is a greyish green powder. It is the strongest of all the powders and is usually mixed with witch hazel. Fullers earth should only ever be used on oily or seborrhoeic conditions. It induces a fast vascular response and is very stimulating. It aids desquamation and has a deep cleansing action.

A combination of these ingredients is mixed with an active liquid ingredient to form a paste. These liquids are as important as the powders and, therefore, should be prescribed with care. They include:

- **Witch hazel** – an astringent, which has a stimulating and drying effect. Used on oily skins.
- **Rose water** – a mild tonic effect. Used on dry skins.
- **Distilled water** – used on normal skin.
- **Orange flower water** – similar to rose water, but slightly stimulating.
- **Vegetable oils** – softening and moisturising effect. Especially good for mature skins and dehydrated conditions.

> **NOTE!** Oil can be warmed prior to mixing. This is particularly good for clients with a mature, dehydrated skin.

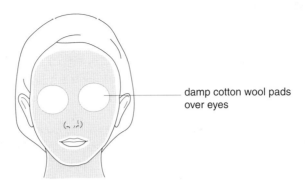

damp cotton wool pads over eyes

Figure 6.19 Applying a face mask

The face mask paste is mixed to a smooth, even consistency and applied to the face and neck using a sterilised brush.

Care should be taken to avoid the hairline, septum, mouth and eyes.

As the mask dries the moisture in the formulation evaporates and has a tightening effect on the skin. Impurities are brought to the surface of the skin and the clay powder absorbs excess oil and removes surface adhesions.

Once the mask has dried, it should be removed using warm water and sponges. Once all trace of the mask has been removed, the skin should be wiped over with dampened cotton wool.

Peel off masks

Peel off masks have become increasingly popular. They are not as strong as clay-based masks. Peel off masks fall into two categories: those based upon waxes (paraffin wax), gums, latex and plastic resins and gel-based ones.

They may be water-based or, for quicker drying, may contain alcohol. They are applied in their liquid state and left to dry on the skin.

This group of masks are easier to apply than clay masks and are gentler on the skin. The wax and latex based products form an occlusive seal on the skin which induces heat and increases the surface moisture on the skin. The effect on the skin is cleansing and, through the creation of heat, promotes an erythema (slight redness). They are suitable for all clients except those who are very sensitive or who have a couperose skin. Gel-based masks are cooling and slightly astringent. Peel off masks are designed to be lifted off the skin when dry, taking softened surface adhesions off the skin.

Non-setting masks
Biological masks

Non-setting masks are usually cooling and refreshing on the skin. They have different effects depending on the type of preparation used. Biological masks are those based on wholly natural ingredients such as herbs, vegetables, fruits, flowers and plant extracts. They are applied in a light film over the skin. This does not harden but becomes firm and drier depending on the binding agent, for example honey.

Biological ingredients can be sliced, chopped up and pulped and placed directly onto the skin or onto a gauze to aid removal. The ingredients may be mixed with honey, cream, egg white or yoghurt. This will lessen the astringent effect of some ingredients.

Most soft fruits have an acidic reaction on the skin and should be used with care. The enzymatic action of some fruits can soften and remove dead skin cells, but may also sensitise.

Herbs and vegetables can stimulate, balance and tone the skin. Plants can stimulate the circulation. Egg yolk, whipped with honey, has a moisturising effect. Whipped egg white or yoghurt has a drawing, tightening effect on the skin.

Specialised masks

These can be both setting and non-setting. They include:

- **Specialised cream masks** – these are usually part of a professional range which provide retailing opportunities for the therapist.
- **Paraffin wax** – an occlusive mask, particularly effective on mature skin types. Specialised products may be applied to the skin prior to application to enhance the effect.
- **Prescription masks** – usually gel-based. These are a series of active products from which tailor-made masks can be created to suit the needs of the individual.
- **Thermal masks** – these masks either generate heat or require an external heat source.

Heat-generating masks are formed from a paste which is applied over a specialised cream or ampoule. The paste sets and as it hardens, generates heat. The mask is lifted away in a solid form upon cooling.

Heat-reliant masks are preparations which include the use of warmed oil to mix and bind formulations. A gauze is placed over the application and an infra-red lamp may be used to further increase the warmth.

Activity

1 List the uses and effects of a fullers earth mask.

2 What is understood by thermal masks?

3 What is an occlusive mask?

4 What precautions should be taken when using biological masks?

Activity

1 Working with a colleague, design a face mask using biological ingredients.

2 List the formulation and the effect on the skin.

AFTER CARE

This unit has discussed treatments designed to improve the condition of the facial skin. To ensure optimum effectiveness of the treatment, the client should be advised on how to treat the skin between visits for professional facials.

This advice should cover three aspects:
1. General care of skin.
2. Treatment of skin following professional treatment.
3. Other factors.

General care of skin

The client may have been carrying out a particular skin care regime for years. Their routine may require adapting or changing completely. It is quite common to discover that a client's skin care routine is actually the cause of the skin problem. The therapist should ensure that clients are aware that their skin type will not stay the same and that it may go through several changes.

It is very important that the therapist is knowledgeable about the product range available in the salon. You should read all available information, as this will increase your confidence when advising your clients. Most salons stock a professional range. This means that it is a range which can only be purchased through approved salons, it also means, as discussed earlier in this chapter, that there is a selling opportunity for the therapist (see pages 107 and 160). The client will see a better result if the products used in the facial treatment are complemented by professionally prescribed products to use at home.

Treatment of skin

After care advice should also relate to special treatment of the skin following salon treatment. Clients should be advised that any erythema caused by treatment will quickly disperse and is temporary. They should also be told what activities and products to avoid. This will depend on the type of treatment. However, it is wise to recommend that the client avoids using sunbeds, sunbathing, extremes of temperature or using strong scented products. Some facial treatments may carry on working for up to 24 hours and it is important for the client not to irritate the area. Rough handling of the skin or using harsh inappropriate products will only serve to undo the positive effects of the facial.

Other factors

The professional beauty therapy treatment will undoubtedly benefit and improve most skin conditions. It is important though that you consider other factors which may be the underlying cause of a skin problem or may influence the predicted outcome of the treatment.

Stress, for example, is thought to be one of the main causes of premature ageing. It can affect the client's sleeping pattern, can lead to depression, weight loss or gain and sallow dull looking skin. Relaxation activities such as massage could be suggested to help improve the condition.

Smoking will also have an adverse effect on the skin. It can reduce the amount of oxygen reaching the skin, as the blood is polluted by the gases inhaled during smoking. This affects the oxygen reaching the cells and results in dryness and dilated capillaries. It will also cause the formation of premature lines around the lips. It, of course, has other very harmful effects on the rest of the body!

Diet also contributes to healthy skin. There has been a culture of change in dietary habits over the last 20 years. More food allergies, fad dieting and an increase in eating disorders have been seen. There has been a change in eating patterns and a greater reliance on snacks and processed foods. The effects of this change are evident in the increase in nutrition-related problems. A healthy body requires a balanced diet which contains a mixture of proteins, fats and carbohydrates.

Exercise also affects the skin. If the client has a healthy well balanced diet and takes moderate regular exercise they will look and feel better. They will have more energy and be less prone to tiredness and tension.

The therapist must understand the limitations of the professional salon treatment. That it will help to improve the condition, but for how long depends on the client's willingness to bring about an alteration in lifestyle.

ULTRA VIOLET LIGHT AND THE SKIN

The effects of the sun and sunbeds on the skin are well documented. Articles appear each year in journals and magazines just before the summer holidays or the ski season offering wise and precautionary advice. It is important that, as a beauty therapist, you have an awareness and understanding of the long term effects of exposure to sunlight.

Ultra violet rays are damaging to the skin, although some types are more harmful than others. The amount of damage can be directly attributed to the length of time spent exposed to the ultra violet rays. Damage can range from mild irritation to blistering, swelling and inflammation. Continued exposure to sunlight can cause permanent damage to the skin. The most severe and increasingly common danger is that of **melanoma** – skin cancer. Fair skinned people are particularly prone to melanoma.

The colour of skin, as discussed earlier in this unit (see page 155), can be attributed to the amount of melanin present in the skin. The darker the skin the higher the melanin content. Melanin protects the skin from the effects of sunlight. Therefore, darker skins are less prone to conditions such as melanoma and have more tolerance to ultra violet exposure. It should be noted, however, that all skin types will suffer from the effects of over-exposure: excessive dryness and premature formation of wrinkles.

The skin becomes drier following exposure to ultra violet light and eventually the collagen fibres, which give the skin its elasticity, break up. This is exactly the same process that occurs during ageing. It is the prolonged exposure which speeds this process up, resulting in premature ageing. The effects of ultra violet exposure cannot be reversed.

Psoriasis and acne are the only conditions which can be improved through controlled exposure to sunlight. This works by causing the surface of the skin to peel slightly, unblocking the sebaceous glands and increasing desquamation (removal of skin cells).

Sunscreens

The client should always be advised to use a sunscreen. These products have a **sun protection factor** (SPF) which indicates the length of time the skin can be exposed to the sun, following application. Factors to consider when selecting a sunscreen are the type of skin and the type of activity to be carried out, for example swimming, skiing, etc.

If the product had an SPF of 3 the wearer could stay in the sun three times longer than normal without burning.

- Very fair skins which burn easily   use SPF 20/25+
- Fair skins which burn after 10 minutes   use SPF 10+
- Skin which tans easily   use SPF 2+

Fake tanning products

The known effects and dangers of the sun still fail to dissuade some clients. It may be prudent for the therapist to recommend fake tanning products. These used to be hard to apply, had a dreadful odour and invariably dried streaky. More recently, these products have become refined, effective and pleasantly scented! The professional application of these products has become a very popular service offered by the beauty therapist.

The skin should always be exfoliated and a light application of moisturiser applied. The skin should then be allowed to settle for a few minutes prior to applying the self-tanning product. Two or three light applications should be made to avoid streaking. The client should be advised to reapply after a few hours depending upon the depth of colour required. When applying to areas of the skin prone to dryness such as knees and elbows, a small amount of moisturiser should be mixed with the self-tanning product.

It is important for the therapist to wash her hands thoroughly after application and the client should also be advised if they are going to use the product at home.

Most fake tans contain dihydroxyacetone. This adheres to the keratin cells and stains them an orangey-brown. As the skin desquamates the stained cells are shed resulting in a gradual fading of the tan.

UNIT 7

Remove and lighten hair using temporary methods

In this unit you will learn about:

- the basic principals of hair growth
  - the structure of hair
  - types and colour of hair
  - terminology
- preparing the work area for temporary hair removal
  - selecting products and materials for depilatory treatments
  - safety precautions
  - preparing the client for treatment
  - assessing clients and preparing a treatment plan
  - various methods of temporary hair removal
  - treatment methods for different areas of the body
  - erythema cause and treatment
  - aftercare advice
  - care and maintenance of equipment
- lightening hair using bleaching techniques
  - preparation
  - procedure.

INTRODUCTION

Depilation is the removal of superfluous hair using **temporary methods**. The hair is plucked from the follicle but the base of the follicle (the **papilla**) remains intact and can therefore provide nourishment for a new hair to grow. Temporary hair removal only lasts for two to six weeks depending on the individual.

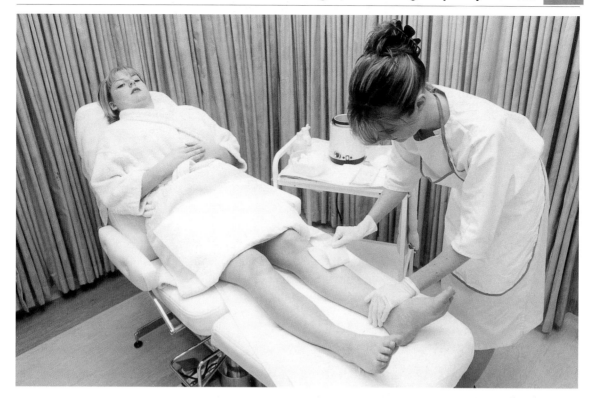

Depilation uses a range of methods which pluck or pull the hairs from the skin:
- hot wax
- cool wax
- hand sugaring
- strip sugaring
- tweezing.

If hair is removed **permanently** using an electrical current or laser, this is called **epilation**. Sometimes hair on the arms or face is treated by **lightening the hair** using bleaching products instead of removing it. This technique is discussed later in the unit.

HAIR STRUCTURE AND GROWTH

Hair is a dead, keratinised structure protruding out of an indentation in the skin called a **follicle**. It can be divided into two portions:

1. The **hair shaft** – the part which extends above the surface of the skin.
2. The **hair root** – the part below the surface of the skin.

There are two main classifications of hair:

1. **Vellus hair** is the soft, downy hair found all over the body except the eyelids, lips, palms of hands and soles of the feet. This type of hair originates from a lobe of a

sebaceous gland and so has a shallow follicle. When the follicle is stimulated, for example there is an increase in blood circulation, by hormonal changes during puberty, pregnancy or menopause. It is possible for a vellus hair to become a course, dark terminal hair.

2. **Terminal hair** is deep-seated and extends from a deeper follicle. These hairs are found on the scalp, underarm, eyebrows, pubic regions, arms and legs.

The structure of each hair is divided into three layers:

- cuticle
- cortex
- medulla.

The cuticle

The outermost layer, is composed of overlapping transparent scales. The cuticle of hair protects the layers that lie underneath. When substances such as tint or bleach come in contact with the cuticle, the scales become raised due to the alkalinity of the chemicals. This allows the chemicals to enter into the cortex of the hair.

The cortex

Made of many **micro-fibrils** arranged into bunches to form elongated cells, the cortex makes up the bulk of the hair and gives it strength and elasticity. It is within the cells of this layer that granules of pigment can be found. This gives the hair its colour: melanin produces the brown-black shades and pheomelanin gives the red-yellow shades. The cortex is also where the chemicals of tinting, bleaching and perming have their effects.

The medulla

This layer is not always present particularly in fine hair. When seen it lies in the centre of the cortex and its function is unclear.

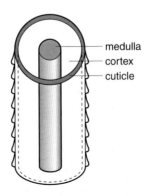

Figure 7.1 Structure of hair

The structure of the hair follicle

The hair follicle is formed by a depression of the epidermis downwards into the dermis to form a tube like structure. It is from this that the hair grows. The lower portion of the follicle is called the **bulb**. Approximately two-thirds of the way up the follicle lies the sebaceous glands which produce sebum, a natural oil. This lubricates the neck of the follicle, the skin surface and the hair.

The bulb

The lower portion of the bulb is called the dermal papilla or matrix. This has a rich blood supply and is where the cells grow and divide by a process called mitosis. New cells are pushed upwards changing shape and becoming keratinised as they do so, until they enter the upper bulb or **keratogenous zone**. Here they harden and form the layers of the hair.

The dermal papilla

This is an elevation into the base of the bulb which contains a rich blood supply. It is from here that the cells receive the food and oxygen necessary for mitosis to occur. Whilst the follicle is in contact with the dermal papilla it will be active, in other words producing a hair.

The inner root sheath

The inner root sheath is made up of similar cells to the cuticle of the hair. They lie in the opposite direction, facing down towards the dermal papilla. This allows the two cuticles to interlock helping to secure the hair in its follicle.

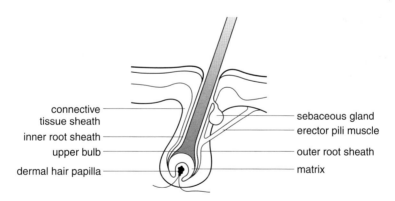

Figure 7.2 A hair follicle

The outer root sheath

The outer root sheath is continuous with the stratum germinativum of the epidermis and is therefore made up of growing cells (**hair germ cells**). This enables the follicle to grow and renew cells during the life cycle. The root sheath can be clearly seen as a silver sheath on some hairs when they are plucked from the follicle.

Activity

Look closely at the hairs you remove on the waxing strip and you will see some with a silver sheath. Others have no sheath, but a black blob on the end. Some hairs may appear straight across at the root as if they have been cut. They may have broken off.

The way the root looks can identify the stage in the life cycle of each hair. Turn to page 000 to read about the life cycle of hair.

LIFE CYCLE OF HAIR

A hair follicle actively produces hair for distinct periods of time, before going through stages of change and then rest. There are three stages that a follicle goes through:
1. **anagen** – the active, growing stage
2. **catagen** – the changing stage
3. **telogen** – the resting stage.

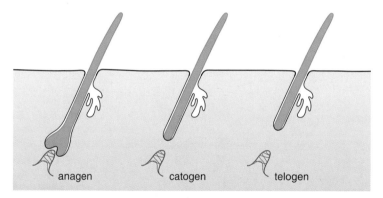

Figure 7.3 The three stages in the life cycle of a hair

Anagen

At the onset of anagen, the hair germ cells in the outer root sheath are stimulated into activity by hormones. This results in the formation of the **dermal cord**. The cells of the dermal cord undergo mitosis and a new follicle is produced. This grows in length and width, the food and oxygen being obtained from the connective tissue sheath. The newer follicle extends downwards to the dermal papilla which enlarges and the bulb is formed around it. The bulb begins production of new hair cells, receiving the necessary nourishment from the dermal papilla. These cells form the inner root sheath and then a new hair. As the new hair grows up the follicle, it may push the old hair out (if it has not fallen out already) and eventually the new hair appears at the surface. The hair continues to grow whilst the follicle is active. This varies according to the area of the body but can be as long as six years. Towards the end of anagen, melanin production begins to slow down and eventually ceases as the follicle enters the next stage.

Catagen

This stage is also known as the transitional stage where the dermal papilla breaks down and the hair detaches itself from the base of the follicle and the bulb. The hair is known as a **club hair** because of its appearance. When plucked it has a black bob on the end. Club hairs are only attached to the follicle by the inner root sheath. The hair continues to rise up the follicle to just below the sebaceous gland until it is no longer attached by the inner root sheath. At this time the hair can be removed from the follicle just by brushing. The follicle below the hair shrinks and breaks away from the dermal papilla but the remaining cells are already organising themselves to form the new matrix and hair germ cells. All this takes place over a period of a few days.

Telogen

Known as the resting stage, the follicle remains at approximately half of its normal length for a few weeks before anagen begins again.

Knowledge of the hair growth cycle is important to a beauty therapist for waxing. It can explain the premature appearance of hairs after waxing and the difference in time between treatments as well as being able to judge the effectiveness of an epilation treatment.

SELF ASSESSMENT TEST

1. Name the three layers of the hair.
2. In which layer of the hair do tinting, bleaching and perming have an effect?
3. What is the function of the inner root sheath?
4. What is the name given to cell division?
5. Where in the follicle does cell division take place?
6. What is the name given to the active growing stage of the hair life cycle?
7. How long does this stage last?
8. Which part of the follicle produces hair germ cells?
9. What is the name given to the resting stage of hair growth?
10. What is a club hair?

Element 7.1

Assess clients and prepare treatment plans

NOTE! For further information on this element see page 153.

CLIENT CONSULTATION AND TREATMENT PLANNING

A knowledge of the techniques and their application is essential before embarking on hair removal or lightening.

A consultation should be carried out before every treatment to establish:
1. contraindications
2. the client's expectations of the treatment
3. the amount, type and area of hair growth.

When assessing the client for treatment you will discuss the client's requirements and examine the area to be treated. Begin by checking for contraindications and examining the condition of the skin and hair. Note the length, texture, colour and growth pattern of the hair. This will help you decide on the method of treatment and, if waxing, the direction in which the wax is to be applied.

Some clients can be very sensitive to the products so it is important to check the record card to see if she has had hair removal or lightening treatment previously and whether the skin reacted in any way. New clients should be questioned carefully to establish whether they have had any previous adverse reaction to treatment.

The treatment should be clearly explained to the client, giving some indication of how it might feel and how the skin may react and look for a short while afterwards. The normal skin reaction can be a shock to some clients who expect smooth skin immediately.

Skin reaction from waxing
Normal reaction
The following may occur after waxing and are quite normal reactions:
- erythema in the area

- slight swelling
- tiny red spots around the hair follicles
- blood spots may appear during under arm or bikini line waxing – this is due to the coarse nature of the hair and follicles which have a rich blood supply
Normal reactions will last anything from a few minutes to several hours depending on the area treated and the skin type.

Abnormal skin reaction

The following signs should concern you:

- erythema or red spots on the skin which persists for more than a few hours
- irritation, which may be an indication of an allergic reaction
- burning sensation accompanied by excessive erythema and possibly swelling
- bruising can occur when a poor technique is used – for example pulling the wax upwards especially on the bikini line or on clients with loose crêpe skin.

Skin reaction from sugaring

Sugaring is regarded as a more gentle method of hair removal providing benefits to the skin such as softening and smoothness. There is very little erythema following treatment and the red spots which often appear after waxing are reduced. There may be an increase in ingrown hairs for those clients who are prone to the condition.

SUPERFLUOUS HAIR

Superfluous hair (unwanted hair), usually found under the arm, bikini line and legs, is regarded by some western societies as unattractive and unacceptable on the female. Many European women, on the other hand, do not regard this as a problem and do not remove hair from under-arm or legs.

Smooth, flawless skin is much sought after, particularly during the summer when the body is more exposed or when clients are going on holiday. It is then that waxing becomes a very popular salon treatment. There are also client's who have waxing all the year round.

The amount and colour of superfluous hair will vary in individuals but is regarded as normal if it follows a normal growth pattern on the legs, underarm and bikini line, and can be seen as a family characteristic like, for example, fair skin or blue eyes. Superfluous hair, however, may be unsightly because it is dark or grows thickly. This can cause embarrassment to the client and she may look to you for appropriate treatment.

For hair removal, the client may use a whole range of home treatments including:

- shaving using an electric or wet razor – this cuts the hair at the surface of the skin leaving a blunt end which will grow through in 24 to 48 hours as rough stubble.
- depilatory cream – this is made up of strong alkaline chemicals which dissolve the

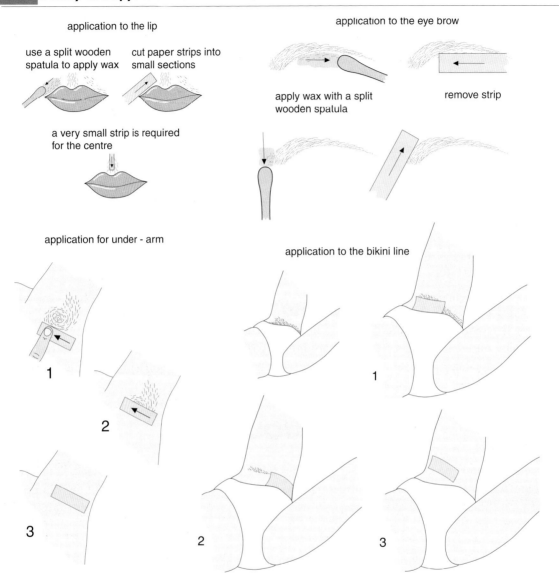

application to the lip

use a split wooden spatula to apply wax

cut paper strips into small sections

a very small strip is required for the centre

application to the eye brow

apply wax with a split wooden spatula

remove strip

application for under - arm

1

2

3

application to the bikini line

1

2

3

Figure 7.4 Diagrams to show areas of superfluous hair growth and the direction of hair growth in each case

keratin in the hair and skin. The skin can become very sensitive after application. The hair is only removed to the surface of the skin so will reappear in 24 to 48 hours.

■ abrasive gloves or a pumice stone which is rubbed over the skin in circular movements. This breaks off the hair at the surface of the skin.

■ clipping or cutting may be used to cut hairs from moles (which should not be waxed or plucked) or to cut the hair close to the surface of the skin. A course stubble would be the result.

■ home waxing kits in the form of pre-waxed strips or roll on wax are applied in the usual way to pull the hairs from the follicle. Home waxing can be very messy and the backs of the legs and underarms can be very difficult to reach.

DEPILATORY WAXING PRODUCTS

Waxing

Hot wax has been popular for many years and there are still clients who prefer hot wax, particularly those with dark course hair. However, new products referred to as warm wax which do not require heating to such a high temperature are more popular and in many ways are more economical and hygienic.

Hot wax

Hot wax is mainly beeswax with resin added to make it more pliable. The wax may be a natural amber colour or have colour added to distinguish the product from those of other manufacturers. Sun bleached beeswax is used by some manufacturers to increase the plasticity of the wax. This product is usually opaque and coloured pale pink or lilac.

Beeswax liquefies when heated which allows the wax to be applied to the area using a spatula or brush. The wax coats each hair and as it cools the wax contracts around the hair. The strip of wax is then pulled from the skin.

Warm wax

Warm wax is supplied in tins or plastic containers which can be placed directly into a heater.

The product is mainly synthetic resins which are either water or oil soluble. Additives such as honey improve the sticky property of the wax. Warm wax may be a clear amber colour or be opaque and coloured depending on the manufacturer. The properties of the waxes are similar to beeswax and work by coating the hair with the very sticky substance which is removed using a fabric (calico) or paper strips.

Sugaring techniques

The art of sugaring to remove hair from the body has been passed down by generations from very early times. The technique originates in the Middle East where it was the tradition to remove all the hair from the body of the bride before her wedding day. All the female members of the family would gather to prepare the sugar paste from a recipe which included sugar, water and lemon juice boiled together to a caramelised paste. The sugar was applied as a ritual to ensure that the bride's skin was perfectly smooth.

Sugar paste is now made commercially and can be obtained from wholesalers at a reasonable price. Traditional practitioners of sugaring may make their own paste using a special recipe but this requires considerable experience because of the dangers involved in boiling sugar.

ADVANTAGES AND DISADVANTAGES OF TEMPORARY HAIR REMOVAL METHODS

Advantages

- large areas can be treated
- instant results
- relatively low cost
- usually only slight discomfort to the client.

Disadvantages

- some clients have problems with ingrown hairs
- needs to be repeated at regular intervals
- there is a belief that hair growth increases due to the stimulation of the blood supply to the follicle.

ADVANTAGES AND DISADVANTAGES OF PERMANENT HAIR REMOVAL

Electrical epilation using **short wave diathermy** or **The Blend** (combining short wave diathermy and galvanic currents) are the most commonly used methods for removing hair permanently. Each hair follicle is treated individually and the treatment is generally used for small areas of abnormal hair growth (**hypertrichosis**). This treatment is suitable for facial hair, although some clients may request epilation to treat the bikini line or legs. However, this can be expensive and time consuming.

Advantages

- once an area has been successfully treated it will remain free from hair (unless new growth as a result of hormone changes occurs)
- regrowth of hairs may occur after a follicle has been treated but these will be finer in texture.

Disadvantages

- skin reaction may occur
- some discomfort or even pain may be experienced by the client when working on sensitive areas such as the upper lip or around the nose
- there is a high cost involved if large areas are to be treated
- treatment by poorly trained or incompetent therapists can lead to permanent skin damage, such as scarring.

CONTRAINDICATIONS TO WAXING AND SUGARING

1. Specific to the area to be waxed

Waxing and sugaring should not be carried out if there is evidence of skin disease or infection in the area to be treated –

- chin or lip wax: herpes simplex (cold sores)
- eyebrows: eye infection such as conjunctivitis.

2. Medical conditions

Do not carry out waxing or sugaring on the following areas if these medical conditions are present:

- legs: varicose veins, very thin or loose skin, oedema
- underarm: mastitis or if the client has had a mastectomy.

3. General

Some other contraindications are:

- sun burn
- recent scar tissue
- cuts, abrasions, open sores such as bites or stings
- hairy moles, raised lesions such as warts
- hypersensitivity
- inflammation or swelling.

> **NOTE!** Diabetes is a contraindication to sugaring because of the possibility of absorbing the product through the skin. Waxing may be used with permission from the client's doctor. You must be particularly careful to ensure that the skin does not over react to treatment. Some people may be allergic to waxing products causing extreme erythema and irritation.

Element 7.2

Prepare the work area and client for treatments

PREPARATION FOR WAXING AND SUGARING

Equipment and materials

The following things are needed:

- large secure trolley
- couch prepared with plastic sheeting and/or disposable bed paper (towels and sheets should not be used as the various wax products can be difficult to remove from bed linen)
- heater with sufficient wax or sugar for the treatment (it is recommended that sugar paste is initially heated in a microwave)
- surgical spirit
- cotton wool
- tissues
- talc
- tweezers placed in disinfectant
- soothing lotion
- fabric or paper strips for warm wax and strip sugaring treatment
- palettes for used wax/sugar paste/strips
- a bowl of water or small wet towel is required to wipe your hands when sugaring
- disposable wooden spatulas for waxing and a metal spatula for strip sugaring.

Hygiene, health and safety when waxing and sugaring
Heating

It is essential that you prepare the wax or sugar paste well in advance of the client arriving. If the salon uses a range of products for different hair types or areas of the body then these must all be ready for use. The client may be annoyed if she arrives for depilation treatment to find that she has to wait for the wax or sugar paste to heat to the correct temperature or for it to cool to the working temperature because the heater has been left on.

Hot wax requires a thermostatically controlled stainless steel unit to which blocks or pellets of beeswax are added. The wax must be allowed to melt slowly to a working temperature of around 48°C, which will take approximately 40 minutes. Overheating, which can destroy the

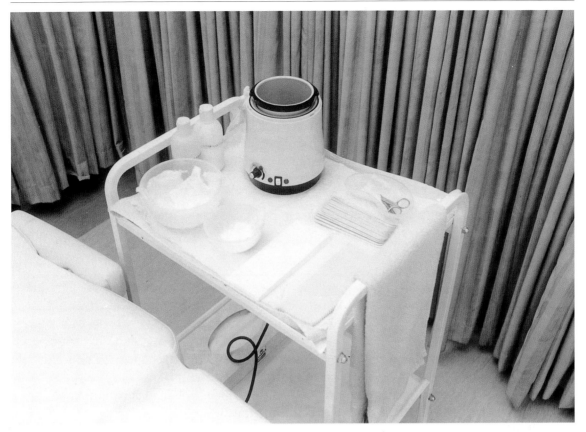

Figure 7.5 Equipment for waxing

properties of the wax, must be avoided. Hot wax is usually a pale amber colour, but darkens as it is heated especially if it is allowed to overheat.

All wax heaters should be thermostatically controlled. However, it is sometimes necessary to boost the temperature whilst working to keep the correct consistency of the wax. The consistency of the wax is an indication of the temperature. If the wax is thick like toffee it is not heated sufficiently and will be impossible to apply to the area evenly. If, on the other hand, the wax is giving off fumes or smoke, it is an immediate indication of overheating and it cannot be used until cool. If overheated, the wax will be very runny and impossible to control on the spatula. Modern hot wax machines do not have the filtering mechanism of earlier equipment. This is because it is now considered unacceptable to reuse wax, by filtering out hairs. To ensure that there is no risk of cross infection, all waxing materials must be disposed of after each client. This includes spatulas, used wax etc.

Warm wax (sometimes called strip wax or cool wax) will usually require heating to a temperature of 35–45°C although some products are applied cold. The wax may be heated in its own container in an especially designed thermostatically controlled unit. A more recent method encloses the wax in a cartridge with a roller type applicator which is disposed of after use.

Whatever the product or method, it is important that you follow the manufacturers instructions. Warm wax can overheat and there is a risk of burning the client. The heating must be controlled carefully, in the same way as for hot wax. There are safety precautions for heating and testing the temperature (see page 204).

Sugaring paste will require heating to a working temperature using a microwave or a thermostatically controlled heater. The paste must be heated gently and allowed to stand for 5 minutes before using. When using a microwave to heat the container of paste, it will require only 1–2 minutes on full power to heat to the required temperature. Leave to stand to allow the heat to distribute evenly through the paste.

Because the sugar paste retains heat, it can be moved to the trolley where it will stay at a working temperature for some time, or the container of paste can be kept in a hot water bath to help retain the temperature for longer.

> **NOTE!** Always follow the manufacturer's instructions.

Hygiene procedures

- The work area should be prepared with clean disposable paper and plastic sheeting.
- Spatulas and wax strips should be disposed of after use.
- Hot wax must be disposed of after each client to limit the risk of cross infection.
- The area of skin to be waxed must be cleansed with surgical spirit.
- Tweezers should be placed in disinfectant.
- Remember to wash your hands before and after treatment.

Safety precautions

1. Waxing

- Wax which has been heated should not be moved around the salon.
- Wax heaters must be placed on a secure trolley.
- Heaters must have a thermostat to control the heating of the wax.
- Prevent leads from the heater trailing across the floor.
- You should test heated wax on your wrist before applying to the client. Remember to check the consistency of the wax. Overheated wax will be very runny, may emit strong fumes or give off smoke.
- Test the client's tolerance to the heat of the wax (particularly when using hot wax) by applying a small amount with a spatula to an area of the skin on which you will be working.

2. Sugaring

- The safety precautions for waxing apply also to sugaring.
- Sugar paste needs to be heated carefully, especially if using a microwave.
- When using a microwave, remember that the paste will heat from the centre of the container. The outside of the paste may remain cool. Do not be fooled!

- Leave the paste for up to 10 minutes before use.
- Make sure you test the temperature before putting your fingers into the paste when hand sugaring.

PREPARING THE CLIENT

Prepare the client by asking her to remove the necessary items of clothing. She should be allowed privacy and be provided with a gown or towels. Positioning the client for a bikini line wax is not very elegant so you must ensure that some means of cover is available.

Protect the client's clothing using disposable bed paper or old clean towels (wax can spoil towels by getting into the fibres). Sugaring paste is easily removed by laundering the towels.

If you are applying wax to the face, protect the client's hair by placing disposable paper or a towel loosely over her hair.

Prepare the skin by wiping over the area to be treated with cotton wool soaked in surgical spirit. This acts as an antiseptic to cleanse the skin and remove oil and perspiration from the surface of the skin. This must be done thoroughly when sugaring or the paste will not stick to the hairs. An antiseptic solution may be used, especially if the client is allergic to surgical spirit, but it will leave the skin damp. The skin must be allowed to dry before applying the talc. Surgical spirit evaporates immediately making it a more efficient product to use.

Cleansing the skin should be done against the direction of hair growth to help to lift the hairs from the skin. At the same time, you can take note of the direction of the hair growth and plan how the wax needs to be applied. This is particularly important under the arm where the hair tends to grow in a swirl (see diagram on page 212). Effective sugaring, on the other hand, does not depend on the direction of natural hair growth and the paste can be worked in any direction.

Talcum powder is applied for waxing and sugaring using a pad of cotton wool against the hair growth to ensure that the hairs are lifted from the skin.

Element 7.3

Remove unwanted hair to meet client requirements

PROCEDURE FOR WAXING

Hot wax

1. Check the consistency of the wax before testing the temperature on your wrist. If it feels comfortable to you, apply to a small area on the client's skin and check the client's tolerance to the temperature.

2. The correct consistency of wax will enable you to control it on the spatula and apply it to the skin without dripping. Twisting the spatula will control the wax as you take it from the heater across to the client. It is essential that the heater is close by on the side of the couch nearest to your working hand. Do not reach across the client for the wax as it may drip wax on her clothing.

3. Apply the wax **against the direction of hair growth** in organised strips, following the growth pattern of the area. The diagram opposite shows a routine to ensure that the application of the wax is systematic. An adhoc approach will take longer and possibly leave hairs behind.

4. Hot wax needs to be applied thickly. This is done by building up one or two layers quickly, before the wax on the skin is allowed to cool. The aim is to achieve thick edges which can be picked up between the fingers, making it easy to pull off. If the application is too thin, the wax will cool rapidly and be too brittle to remove.

5. The wax can be gently pressed onto the skin as it cools to increase its attachment to the hairs.

6. To remove the wax, flick up the bottom edge of the strip gripping the wax between the thumb and first finger, with the free hand supporting the skin. A long, quick movement is needed to remove the wax. It can be very uncomfortable for the client if, when flicking up the edge or removing the wax, it is done slowly. If the hand is lifted pulling the skin upwards this can cause bruising, particularly in the bikini line area.

7. Pressure should be applied to the area immediately after the wax has been removed. This helps to reduce the stinging effect.

8. As you gain confidence in applying the wax, you will be able to apply a few strips at a time removing them in sequence. This will ensure that the treatment is carried out in a commercially acceptable time of 30 minutes for a half leg wax with additional 15 minutes added for other areas. Variations to timings depend on how course and dense the hair growth is.

9. Any small pieces of wax which remain in the skin can be lifted by using the strip of

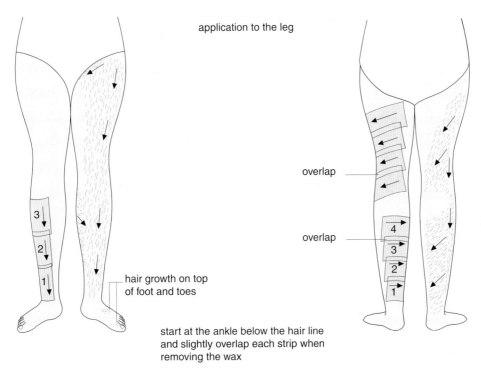

application to the leg

overlap

overlap

3
2
1

4
3
2
1

hair growth on top
of foot and toes

start at the ankle below the hair line
and slightly overlap each strip when
removing the wax

Figure 7.6 Direction of hair growth on legs and strip/warm wax application

wax that has just been removed and pressing on to the area. If pieces are particularly stubborn, dip your finger into the hot wax pan and press it on to the wax remaining on the skin. This should lift it off.

10. If the wax has cooled and become difficult to remove, another layer of hot wax from the heater will soften it sufficiently to aid its removal.

11. Check that the area is free of hair. Odd hairs can be tweezed, but large areas will need a further application of wax. This must be done carefully because the skin will be more sensitive and warm from the previous application. Check with the client that the temperature of the wax is still comfortable before continuing.

12. Apply after wax lotion either by using gentle effleurage massage or by soothing onto the area with the fingers, or with cotton wool for bikini and underarm areas.

It is important to develop a technique which leaves the minimum of wax on the skin. This is achieved by:

- applying several layers of wax
- leaving thick edges to enable the wax to be lifted off in one go
- not allowing the wax to overheat and become brittle
- removing the wax when it is still slightly warm and pliable
- working in a methodical way over the area.

Warm wax

1. Check the consistency of the wax before testing on your skin. Remember if the wax is allowed to overheat, it will become very runny and may give off fumes.
2. Test the wax on the inside of your wrist. If it feels comfortable you can apply a small amount on the client in the area to be treated.
3. Take sufficient wax onto the spatula, scrape one side of the spatula on a bar and hold flat as you move to the client to avoid drips.
4. Apply the wax with the edge of the spatula **following the hair growth** to give a **thin** layer. (Note that this is unlike hot wax which is applied **against** the hair growth in **thick** layers.)
5. The skin must be supported with the free hand to prevent over stretching the skin.
6. Take a fabric or paper strip and press it over the wax. Smooth over firmly with the hand to ensure the wax is sticking to the strip.
7. Grip the bottom edge of the strip with the fingers and pull the strip away very quickly **against** the direction of the hair growth. Stretch and support the skin with the other hand. The strip must be removed parallel to the skin. If the strip is lifted up away from the surface of the skin, it will cause bruising and considerable discomfort to the client.
8. Apply pressure to the area immediately. This helps to reduce the stinging effect which may occur when the strips are removed.
9. The same strip can be used again until it becomes thick with the wax and does not remove the hair. It can be disposed of by folding the wax sides together and placing in a palette or suitable container away from the client. (The client does not want to see the removed hair lying around the work area.)
10. You should aim to work methodically and cleanly.

PROCEDURE FOR SUGARING

Hand sugaring

1. Test the temperature of the paste.
2. Take sufficient paste from the container with the fingers. It should be warm and pliable.

> **NOTE!** The art of sugaring relies on the ability of the practitioner to adjust the paste to the correct consistency. This depends on several factors such as the heat of the hands, the temperature in the room and the climate. Adding a few drops of water using a water spray can alter the consistency dramatically. Selecting a soft paste in winter or a hard paste in the summer can help to achieve the right consistency.

3. Spread the ball of paste on the skin using the middle three fingers in a strip about 6 inches long. When working on the legs or using less paste in smaller areas spread to an appropriate length.
4. The skin must be supported using the free hand (clean hand) by stretching the skin.

5. Remove the paste by flicking back along its length without lifting upwards. The process is repeated quickly on the next area until the paste loses its pliability, becomes full of hair and cools.

> **NOTE!** This technique requires considerable practice. The paste will change from amber to a cream opaque colour as it is worked and cools. The used paste is placed in a palette ready for disposal simply by soaking in hot water. The sugar dissolves leaving the hair which can be disposed of.

Strip sugaring

There are many similarities between warm waxing and strip sugaring techniques.

1. Apply the strip sugar very thinly using a flexible metal spatula in the direction of the hair growth.
2. Remove the strip sugar with fabric strips against the hair growth, supporting the skin below the strip to be removed.
3. Press the hand on the treated area immediately to help to reduce any stinging.

TREATMENT METHODS FOR DIFFERENT AREAS OF THE BODY

Although the majority of hair removal is from the legs and bikini line, the client may request removal of unwanted hair from other areas of the body. This will require a different approach to application and support for the skin. Figure 7.7 illustrates the application methods for different areas.

Bikini line

The skin in this area is very delicate and prone to bruising if too much pressure is applied. It is possible that there will be some bleeding from the follicles. This is because strong course hairs have deeper follicles. Make sure that any cuts or open wounds on your hands are covered by waterproof dressing and a rubber glove is worn on the hand which applies pressure after the wax is removed to protect yourself from infection. Wipe the area to be treated with cotton wool and antiseptic. Dispose of the soiled cotton wool in a closed waste bin. Correct positioning of the client will assist in the easy removal of the hair.

Underarm

Positioning of the client to reveal the whole of the axilla is important. Take special note of the circular direction of hair growth.

Facial including eyebrows, lip and chin

When working on the face, the client's clothing and hair must be protected. The areas to be treated are small, so application must be very careful and neat.

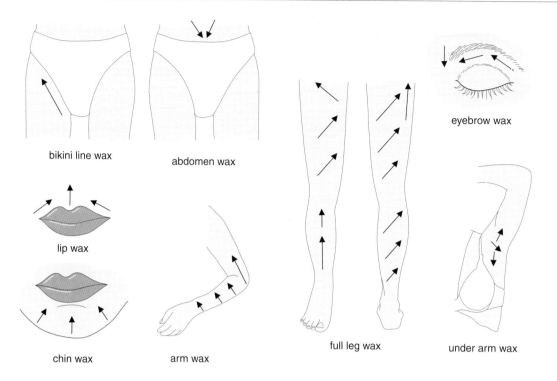

bikini line wax

abdomen wax

eyebrow wax

lip wax

chin wax

arm wax

full leg wax

under arm wax

Figure 7.7 Diagrams to show the wax application methods for different parts of the body

Arms

The arm can be rested on the couch with the client sat on a stool. The hair may be quite long with a tendency to break off if a good technique is not used.

Abdomen

The area is soft making stretching of the skin more difficult. The client should lie flat on the couch to stretch the area as much as possible.

Legs

Leg waxing can be a full leg or up to and including the knee, which is termed half leg. The toes and tops of the feet may also be included. A system of application must be used to avoid missing areas and to work cleanly and efficiently.

Completing treatment and after care

It is important to examine the area you have treated to ensure that all the hairs have been removed and that the treatment meets the client's expectations. If there are just odd hairs which have been missed, these can be removed with tweezers. Larger areas may need a second application, so do not apply any lotions to the skin until you are absolutely sure that the client is satisfied.

If the wax has not removed the hair successfully it could be that:
- the hair was too short for the wax to grip properly
- the area was not cleansed sufficiently to remove body lotion/oil
- warm wax was applied too thickly or allowed to build up on the paper strip
- the wax was applied incorrectly without following the natural hair growth.

Following treatment you should wipe over the area with after wax lotion, depending on the product used:
- **Oil soluble wax** will require an oil-based after wax lotion to remove any traces left on the skin.
- **Water soluble wax** or sugar paste can be removed by wiping over the leg with wet cotton wool and drying with disposable paper or tissue. Some practitioners recommend that sterile water is used (boiled water) to avoid any infection entering the open follicles.
- **Hot wax** tends to leave small particles of wax behind, so the area will require thorough cleansing with suitable after wax lotion or surgical spirit although this can be very harsh on the skin. A soothing cream is massaged onto the skin to cool and moisturise.

This is an ideal opportunity to explain to the client any skin reaction and to give her home care advice.

Home care advice
Explain the skin reaction to the client and that it will take several hours for the skin to return to normal. During the 24 hours after treatment she must avoid the following:
- wearing tight clothing over the treated area, especially the bikini line
- perfumed products such as deodorant
- make up over the area treated on the face – tinted medicated lotion can be used if necessary
- sunbathing, sunbed treatment or hot bath – a warm shower is recommended, followed by a soothing after wax lotion

NOTE! Any skin reaction that lasts longer than 48 hours or progressively becomes worse, for example irritation or erythema, then the client should return to the salon for you to give advice. The most likely explanation will be an allergic reaction to something in the product used. This can be treated with antiseptic soothing lotion and the condition noted on the client's record card.

Infection will appear as pustules at the mouth of the follicle (folliculitis), caused by bacteria entering the open follicle and indicating poor hygiene procedures by the therapist or incorrect home care by the client. This again can be treated by the use of antiseptic lotion. Serious cases may need to be referred to the doctor.

CLEARING AWAY AFTER WAXING

Waxing can be a very messy treatment because of the sticky products used. You must ensure that the area and equipment is cleaned immediately.

The wax heater must be thoroughly cleaned before returning to the store cupboard. Special cleaning products are supplied by the manufacturer, or use warm water for water soluble wax, oil for oil soluble wax and surgical spirit for hot wax. Sugar paste is easily removed with hot water.

Wax heaters should be covered by a lid when cool to ensure that the wax is not left exposed to the air. The warm conditions in the salon can encourage growth of micro-organisms and dust can settle on the surface of the wax. Ensure that there is sufficient wax in the heater before storing. This will save valuable time when you come to reheat the wax for the next client. Wax strips must be disposed of in the waste bin. The plastic bed cover and trolley should be wiped over.

Activity

1 Price the materials and equipment for an individual treatment. Compare the cost of using:
   - sugaring products
   - cool waxing products
   - hot wax.
   Remember the time for treatment will be influenced by the amount of hair, the client's tolerance to the treatment and areas to be treated.

2 Discuss the advantages and disadvantages of each method.

Element 7.4

Lighten hair using bleaching techniques

HAIR LIGHTENING

The purpose of using bleaching products is to lighten dark hair on the face and arms, as a means of disguising hair growth rather than removing the hair. Bleaching lightens the hair by removing natural pigment. The two main pigments in the hair are **melanin** and **pheomelanin** which are deposited in the hair shaft as it grows from the bulb. The amount of colour pigment depends on hereditary factors (family characteristics) and may vary in different parts of the body, for example where the skin and hair is exposed to sunlight the hair will be lighter in colour.

The bleaching process occurs as a result of active ingredients such as **hydrogen peroxide** oxidising the hair pigments. The decolouring of the pigment goes through various stages ranging from black, brown, red, orange, yellow and pale yellow. If, for example, dark hair is bleached and the bleaching cream is removed too soon, the hair may be only at the red or yellow stage. Ideally you will want to achieve a pale yellow result. Dark hair contains more red pigment than light brown hair so requires a longer processing time or stronger bleach to lighten it. It will have a tendency to yellowing, requiring perhaps a further application. Red hair, which is less usual on the body or face, is already light so the client would be unlikely to require bleaching. However, if you were required to bleach red hair, there would be a strong tendency to yellowing because of the amount of natural red pigment in the hair.

The degree of lightening will depend on the strength of the active ingredient and the length of time it is left on. Sometimes the product needs to be reapplied to reach maximum lightness, although the effect on the skin must be taken into account. Redness (erythema) or irritation would prevent any further application. Bleaching will not remove the colour permanently and the hair will become dark again as it grows.

Preparation for bleaching

Cream bleach is normally used because it is thick in consistency and easy to apply. It is important to follow the manufacturer's instructions when using any of the proprietary brands on the market. The hydrogen peroxide is added to activate the cream and it is applied with a small brush or spatula. The hydrogen peroxide, if allowed to come into contact with clothing, towels, and sheets, will remove the colour. It is, therefore, advisable to prepare the couch, trolley and protect the client using disposable paper or white towels.

Assessing the client for treatment

Assess the colour and coarseness of the hair to be bleached and discuss fully with the client the result you expect to achieve. Check for contraindications:

- broken skin
- infection in the area to be treated
- sensitive skin
- dry flaky skin
- sunburn

PROCEDURE FOR BLEACHING

1. Only mix the required amount of bleach. When bleaching the hair on the upper lip, for example, only a small quantity will be required.
2. Prepare the skin by gently wiping over with a cotton wool swab soaked in cold water. The skin in the area to be bleached should not be unnecessarily stimulated prior to application of the bleach.
3. Ensure that the bleach covers the area completely – any gaps will leave dark hairs.
4. The manufacturers instructions will give an indication of the time needed for the bleach to take, but it must be removed immediately if the client experiences any irritation or stinging.
5. Testing the colour can be done during processing by wiping off the bleach in a small area and reapplying as necessary.
6. When the desired result has been achieved the bleach is speedily removed with warm water and cotton wool. Large areas such as the arms may need the bleach to be removed with a spatula prior to using the warm water and cotton wool.
7. It is possible to dry the area and reapply the bleach if the lightening is not satisfactory. However, if the skin shows signs of sensitivity this is not recommended.

After care

The client must be advised to:

- leave her skin free from perfumed products and makeup for 24 hours
- avoid ultra violet light or any form of heat treatment for 24–48 hours
- use soothing lotion such as calamine if there are any signs of redness
- report any adverse reaction to the salon.

SELF ASSESSMENT TEST

1. State two safety measures before applying wax to the client's skin.
2. Give two contraindications specific to the area to be waxed:
   - ■ eyebrows
   - ■ top lip
   - ■ legs.
3. What procedure should be followed to treat the client's skin immediately after waxing.
4. Explain why after shaving the area feels bristly.
5. Hair is bleached using a process called _____ .
6. The active ingredient used in bleaching products is called _____

   _____ .

NOTE! For a Key Skills Task for this unit see page 133.

UNIT 8

Enhance the appearance of the eyebrows and lashes

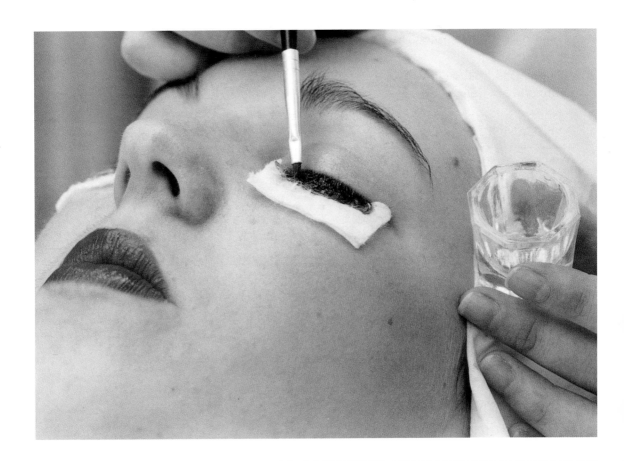

In this unit you will learn about:

- assessing the needs and requirements of the client
- preparing the client for lash and brow treatments
- shaping the eyebrows
- perming the eyelashes
- tinting the brows and lashes
- application of false eyelashes.

INTRODUCTION

The eyes are one of the most sensitive areas of the body. The texture of the surrounding skin is much finer and there is less subcutaneous fatty tissue offering support. Therefore the skin around the eyes can often look darker due to the fine texture and the skin being stretched over a bony prominence in the skull, thus creating a sunken area between the bone and eyeball. No matter how beautiful the facial features are, if the client has dark circles under her eyes or tired eyes or unkempt eyebrows or straight eyelashes the beauty of the other facial features will be detracted. Treatment around the eye area are some of the most important of the salon services and they will have the most dramatic and immediate effect.

PERSONAL APPEARANCE

It is important to ensure your appearance is appropriate (see Unit 1). A professional appearance and manner will instil confidence in the client.

NOTE! Remember to wash your hands before starting any treatment.

Element 8.1
Assess clients and prepare treatment plans

NOTE! For further information on this element see page 103.

ASSESSING THE CLIENT'S NEEDS

The assessment of the client's needs will depend upon the requested treatment. For many treatments around the eye area a **patch test** for sensitivity will be required. Popular salon treatments are tinting brow and lashes, application of semi-permanent eyelashes and one of the most recent developments in eye treatments – eyelash perming.

Patch testing

It is vital that a patch test is carried out at least 48 hours prior to any treatment in the eye area that involves the use of chemical preparations. This should be made clear to the client when they make their appointment. Your salon will have an established procedure for this which will ensure that all staff who take bookings are aware of the policy and can advise the client accordingly. Clients may insist that it is unnecessary as they have their hair tinted or chemically treated before with no ill effect. You must ensure that the client appreciates the sensitivity of the area and that it is common for different areas of the body to be more sensitive than others.

Procedure for patch testing

1. Cleanse an area of skin either behind the ear or in the fold of the elbow.
2. Apply a small amount of the chemical to be used to the area. This may be mixed tint, perm solution or adhesive.
3. Leave for 5 minutes and then wipe over area (if applicable).
4. Advise the client to wash the area if an adverse (or positive) reaction occurs.

Clients should be advised what to expect from a positive reaction: there may be redness, itching and irritation in the area. The client should be told to inform the salon if a positive reaction occurs and to apply a cooling, soothing cream.

> **NOTE!** It is important to note that strong products for wiping/cleansing the area are avoided as the client may be reacting to them rather than the applied treatment product.

The date of the patch test and the outcome (positive or negative) should be recorded on the client's treatment plan or card (see Unit 6).

> **NOTE!** It is important to patch test before **every** treatment as areas with a negative test result can become sensitised between treatments.

EYEBROW SHAPING

Eyebrow shaping is one of the easiest ways of giving definition to the eye area. It is only necessary to remove a few hairs to create a groomed appearance.

Shape of brows

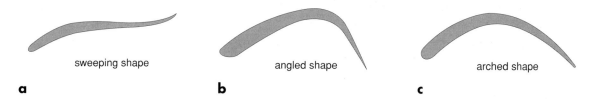

sweeping shape
a

angled shape
b

arched shape
c

Figure 8.1 a b c Corrective eyebrow shapes can be used to give definition to different facial contours

Methods of eyebrow shaping

Eyebrows can be shaped using a variety of methods. They can be waxed using a small spatula and small strip for removal. Care should be taken when waxing such a sensitive area. The skin surrounding the eyes is very thin and delicate. This should be considered prior to using this method.

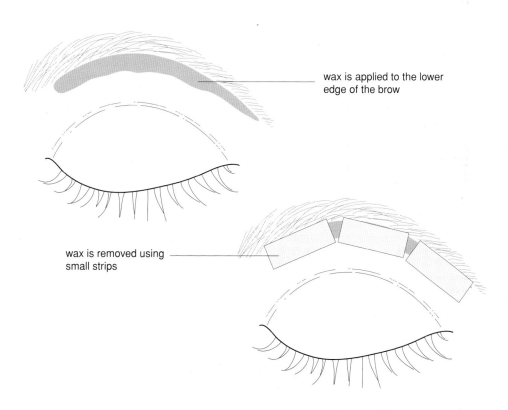

wax is applied to the lower edge of the brow

wax is removed using small strips

Figure 8.2 Waxing eyebrows

Tweezers are the most popular method. There are manual and automatic tweezers available. The automatic tweezer is designed for speed and for removing a lot of hairs.

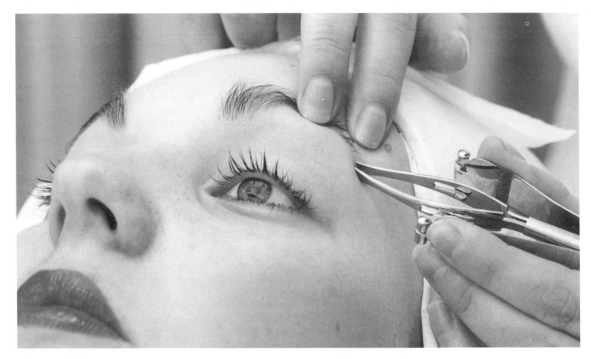

Figure 8.3 Using automatic tweezers

Manual tweezers are used for final shaping and tidying the brows.

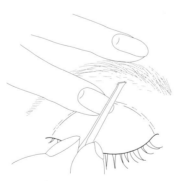

Figure 8.4 Using manual tweezers

15 minutes should be allowed for eyebrow shaping in the treatment schedule.

> **NOTE!** Selection of the tweezer type should be left to the therapist. It is important that you feel confident with the selected tool.

Element 8.2

Prepare the work area and client for eyebrow and lash treatments

Preparation of work station

The couch and trolley should be prepared prior to the client's arrival. There should be clean linen on the couch and the trolley should contain:

- a selection of cleansing and toning products
- a selection of bowls for cotton wool – dry and damp
- tissues
- spatulas
- an eyebrow brush or comb
- witch hazel
- surgical spirit – for wiping tweezers
- tweezers (manual and automatic)
- a hand mirror
- covered waste receptacle
- a steamer or facilities to prepare hot damp cotton wool pads
- treatment plan or record card.

All tools and equipment must be sterilised in the appropriate way and should not be brought to the trolley until they are required for use (see page 17).

Preparation of client

The client should be in a semi-reclining position and the hair and clothing should be protected.

The skin should be cleansed and toned as discussed in Unit 000. It is important to tone to ensure all grease is removed from the area and for client comfort during treatment.

> **NOTE!** Always check for contraindications. Some examples are: sunburn, crepey skin, cuts, bruises etc.

It is important to discuss the desired effect with the client before starting to remove the hairs. Consideration should be given to the natural brow shape and the shape of the client's face. You should also take into account whether the client has had her brows shaped before. If this is the first time it may be wise to shape them gradually over two treatments.

> **NOTE!** Tinting and eyebrow cosmetics can also be used to add definition.

Once the desired outcome has been agreed, the brow area should be brushed against the growth to separate the hairs and then brushed into their natural shape.

Element 8.3
Shape the brows to meet client requirements

PROCEDURE FOR SHAPING THE BROWS

1. The brows should be warmed using either a steamer or hot damp cotton wool pads.
2. The brows should be measured using the following guidelines.

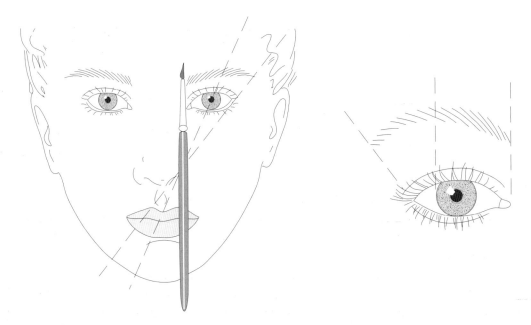

Figure 8.5 Measuring guidelines for eyebrows

3. Hold the skin taut and remove hairs only in the direction of growth.
4. Wipe over constantly with warm damp pads.
5. Brush the brows regularly to ascertain developing shape.
6. Do not work on only one brow. Instead remove a few hairs from each brow to maintain balance.
7. Place removed hairs on a tissue. Do not leave on the skin.
8. When completed wipe over with a witch hazel pad to soothe the area.
9. Show the client the finished result.
10. Provide aftercare advice to avoid application of make-up until the erythema has gone and to wipe over with soothing antiseptic cream.

> **NOTE!** Hairs should only be removed from underneath the brow line. Stray hairs at the temple area or above the brow should only be removed if they do not form part of the main brow growth.

Element 8.4

Tint eyebrows and lashes to meet client requirements

EYELASH AND EYEBROW TINTING

Tinting the eyelashes or brows can be one of the most natural and effective ways of enhancing and defining the eyes. It is particularly popular with clients for whom make-up is prohibited, for those who prefer a more natural look or who are going on holiday and do not want to wear make-up. It can also be effective if the client has changed their hair colour or if they have grey or fair hair and wish to add definition to the eye area. Eyelash tinting is complementary to eyelash perming and application of semi-permanent lashes.

You should allow between 15–20 minutes for eyelash tinting in the treatment schedule and no more than 5 minutes for tinting the brow hairs. This will vary depending upon the client's natural colouring. Those clients who have a lot of red in their hair colour may require a longer processing time to achieve a satisfactory result.

> **NOTE!** Ask the client to refrain from wearing mascara on the day of treatment. This will reduce the possibility of sensitising the area prior to treatment.

Contraindications to lash and brow tinting

It is important to check for contraindications before tinting the eyelashes or brows. Contraindications include:

- positive reaction to the patch test
- cuts and abrasions in the area
- bruised (black eye) eye area
- conjunctivitis
- water eyes
- styes
- inflammation or swelling
- allergy to cosmetics.

Preparation of work station

The work station should be prepared prior to the client's arrival. The couch should have clean linen and the trolley should be prepared with:

- a selection of bowls – for damp and dry cotton wool
- tissues
- a selection of cleansing and toning products
- petroleum jelly
- a small glass or non-metallic dish
- a selection of eyelash tints
- preformed tinting shields
- 10 volume (3 per cent) peroxide

> **NOTE!** It is very important to ensure that the bottle of peroxide is kept tightly closed to maintain the strength of the peroxide.

- orange wood sticks
- small brush
- spatulas
- eyebath and distilled water (for emergencies)
- a covered waste receptacle
- treatment plan or record card.

All tools and equipment should be sterilised in the appropriate way (see page 17).

Preparation of client

The client should be comfortably seated on the couch with her hair and clothing protected. The skin should be cleansed and toned as discussed in Unit 6, or a full cleanse carried out if part of a facial.

You must confirm that the client has had a patch test. You should establish and record the outcome of the test before proceeding with the treatment. The desired effect should be discussed and you should inform the client of your recommendations. You must always consider the different effects and depths of colour achieved by the various tints, depending upon the client's natural colouring.

The client should be informed that, if at any time during the treatment, discomfort (a tingling or burning sensation) is felt, they should inform you immediately.

> **NOTE!** If the client does experience any contra-actions to treatment, the tint should be removed immediately and the eyes rinsed using an eyebath and distilled water.

Procedure for tinting the eyelashes

1. Place the preformed tint shield under the lower lashes. It is advisable to coat the underside with petroleum jelly to help adhesion of the shield.
2. Using a clean, fine brush apply petroleum jelly to the upper eyelid and underneath the lower lashes.

> **NOTE!** The client may have fallen asleep during the process and could open the eyes if suddenly disturbed. It is therefore important to talk generally to the client, explaining each step in the procedure. It is also recommended that you inform the client not to open the eyes until instructed to.

3. The tint should now be mixed.

The formulation is usually 5–6 mm of tint to 2–3 drops of 10 volume peroxide (the tint comes out of a tube rather like toothpaste – you will need to squeeze 5–6 mm long). However, you should always refer to the manufacturer's instructions.

> **NOTE!** Do not mix the tint until the client has been prepared. The tint will start working immediately and if it is not applied straight away the effect will be lessened. Always mix the tint formulation using an orange wood stick. Never use the applicator brush to mix as the tint will clog at the top of the brush head.

4. Apply the tint to the lashes on both eyes using a small sterilised dry brush. The application can be with the eyes open or closed depending upon the client preference.
5. Place warm dampened (not wet!) cotton wool pads over the tint to create warmth. This will assist in the development of the tint and will also help to prevent the client opening their eyes during the processing time.

> **NOTE!** Care must be taken when applying the petroleum jelly. This will act as a barrier between the tint and the skin. However, it will also act as a barrier to the tint if it comes into contact with the hair preventing the tint working on the lashes.

6. The tint should be removed following the manufacturer's recommended processing time. This is normally around 10 minutes.
7. The pad of cotton wool and the tint shield should be grasped and removed in a quick downward movement. This is carried out on both eyes.
8. Dampened cotton wool pads are then used to wipe the lashes. The area should be wiped until the cotton wool shows no evidence of any remaining tint.
9. The client should now be asked to open the eyes. Using a folded, dampened cotton wool pad gently wipe the base of the lashes. Continue until the pad wipes clean.
10. Wipe over the eye area with tonic to remove the petroleum jelly and show the client the finished result.

> **NOTE!** Make sure that you take the tint application as close to the roots as possible. Use a clean finger to gently lift the underside of the eyebrow to expose the roots of the lashes. This is particularly important in both the application and the removal process.

PROCEDURE FOR TINTING THE BROWS

1. The brows should be brushed thoroughly to lift and separate them.
2. Petroleum jelly is applied to the surrounding area, taking care not to touch the hairs that are to be tinted.
3. The tint should be mixed following the same procedure for the lashes.
4. The tint is then applied to both brows using a sterilised small brush. Take care to apply only to the hair and not the skin, or a false look will result.
5. After 1 minute the tint should be checked. This is done by removing a little tint from the inner corners of the brows.

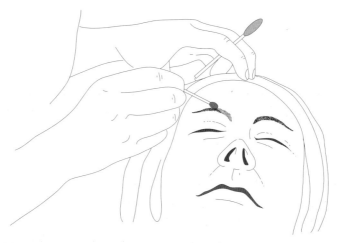

Figure 8.6 Tinting the eyebrows

6. Reapply the tint as necessary, but only leave for 30 to 60 seconds to prevent the colour developing too dark. A slow and gradual build up of colour produces the most natural effect.
7. The tint should be removed as before using clean dampened cotton wool pads.
8. The area should then be wiped over with tonic pads to remove all traces of the petroleum jelly.

> **NOTE!** The brows must not be shaped beforehand and on the same day as tinting. The area will become sensitised following the shaping procedure and the application of tint could cause irritation. The client could have the brows shaped after the tint or could book a shape for the next salon visit.

EYELASH PERMING

This is a new technique which is becoming a very popular salon treatment. It has revolutionised eyelash enhancement and is particularly effective for those with very straight lashes or those want a natural look whilst still defining the eyes. It is also popular with clients who participate in sporting activities. The eyelash perm lasts for 6 to 8 weeks.

The same principles apply as for perming the hair. The perming chemicals are strong and can damage the delicate eye area if they are used incorrectly. It is important, therefore, to refer to manufacturer's instructions.

Contraindications to eyelash perming
- positive reaction to the patch test (using the perm solution)
- inflammation of the eye
- excessively watery eyes
- stye
- conjunctivitis
- cuts and abrasions
- very dry skin.

> **NOTE!** The lashes can be tinted prior to perming to enhance the finished effect of the treatment.

Procedure for eyelash perming
1. The lashes should be clean and free from grease.
2. The lashes are combed and separated.
3. A small roller is secured to the base of the eyelid and the lashes are eased and curled onto the roller.

> **NOTE!** The perm rollers are available in different sizes. These rollers are 'sticky' and a water soluble adhesive is applied to fix the lashes onto the roller.

4. The perm solution is then applied to the lashes and is left to process for 7 to 15 minutes.
5. A neutralising product is then applied and left to develop.
6. The lashes are then wiped over with damp cotton wool and a moisturising lotion is applied to the lashes.

Element 8.5

Apply false eyelashes to meet client requirements

FALSE EYELASHES

These are used for fashion, photographic and catwalk make-ups. They are particularly useful for enhancing short or sparse lashes. They are made from natural hair or nylon and there are two types:

■ temporary
■ semi-permanent

Temporary

These are preshaped lashes on a flexible strip which are applied to the edge of the eyelid. A special latex-based adhesive is used to adhere the lashes to the skin.

Semi-permanent

Available as individual or clusters of three or four flared lashes held together by a fine knot. These are applied to the natural lash using a special adhesive.

> **NOTE!** The client should always be patch tested prior to application of semi-permanent lashes as the adhesive fumes may irritate.

Contraindications

- sensitive or sensitised eyes
- reaction to patch test of bonding adhesive (semi-permanent lashes)
- swollen or inflamed lids
- eye infections.

Procedure for applying temporary lashes

1. Apply small amount of adhesive to a spatula.
2. Using tweezers, gently pick up the strip of eyelashes. Care should be taken to pick up from the centre of the lash side.
3. Stroke the base of the strip through the adhesive so there is a fine line of adhesive along its length.

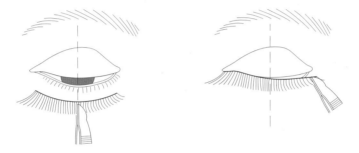

Figure 8.7 Applying temporary eye lashes

4. Lift the brow area to gently pull back the lid. This allows close application to base of the natural lashes.
5. Line tweezers with the centre of the eyelid and gently press strip into place on the closed eye.
6. Secure the inner and outer corners of the strip.
7. Repeat for the other eye.
8. Using clean mascara brush, blend the false and natural lashes together.

At least 10 minutes should be allowed for the application of temporary lashes in the treatment schedule.

Procedure for removing temporary lashes

1. Hold eyelid taut and gently pull away from the outer edge.
2. Remove adhesive from strip.
3. Wipe over natural lashes with mild toner.

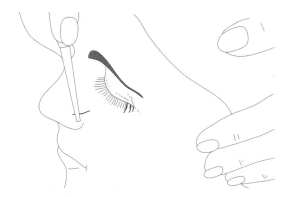

Figure 8.8 Applying semi-permanent lashes

Procedure for applying semi-permanent lashes

1. Ensure natural lashes are clean and free from any oil, which may prevent the adhesive from sticking.
2. Using tweezers, carefully remove lashes individually from the pack and arrange on a tissue. The lashes should be facing away from you.
3. Apply a small amount of adhesive onto a spatula.
4. Raise the client's head slightly.
5. Pick up a lash and dip the knotted end into the adhesive.
6. Ask the client to lower her eyes, but **not** to close them.
7. Lift the brow area to release the fold of skin from the base of the natural lashes.
8. Place the false lash over a natural lash. Stroke gently along its length and locate according to desired outcome.
9. Work alternately between each eye to ensure balance.

> **NOTE!** Always grab the flare, not an individual hair, as this will cause distension to the knot and spoil the lash.

Allow at least 20 minutes for the application of semi-permanent lashes in the treatment schedule.

Procedure for removing semi-permanent lashes

1. Place dampened cotton-wool pads beneath the eyes.
2. Using special solvent or oily eye make-up remover, apply to false lash with a cotton bud.
3. Wait a few seconds and gently ease the lash off.
4. Wipe over with mild toner.

> **NOTE!** Recommend that the client returns to the salon for removal of lashes. Avoid oily products around the eyes as the oil will loosen the adhesive!

SELF ASSESSMENT TEST
1. Why is it important to patch test a client?
2. List the treatments that require a patch test.
3. How can you minimise client discomfort during a brow shape?
4. What advice would you give to a client wanting her eyebrows tinted and shaped?
5. What general guidelines should you use for producing an eyebrow shape?
6. Should a client with excessively dry skin have her eyelashes permed.

Activity

Research trends in eyebrow and eye enhancement over the last four decades. Consider particularly brow shapes and eye definition. Use diagrams and cuttings to support your findings.

NOTE! For a Key Skills Task for this unit see page 133.

UNIT 9

Improve the appearance and condition of nails and adjacent skin

In this unit you will learn about:

- preparing the work area for manicure and pedicure treatment
  - tools and equipment
  - products and materials
  - hygiene procedures
  - preparation of the client
  - health and safety
  - codes of practice
- the structure of nails
  - nail growth
  - nail shapes
  - nail disorders and disease
  - bones and blood supply to hands and feet
  - muscles of the arm and leg
  - lymph drainage of arm and leg
  - nerves of arm and leg
- Assessing client needs by preparing a treatment plan
  - client consultation
  - types of treatments
  - contraindications
  - after care advice
  - client records
- manicure and pedicure treatment methods
  - salon requirements–pricing–timing.

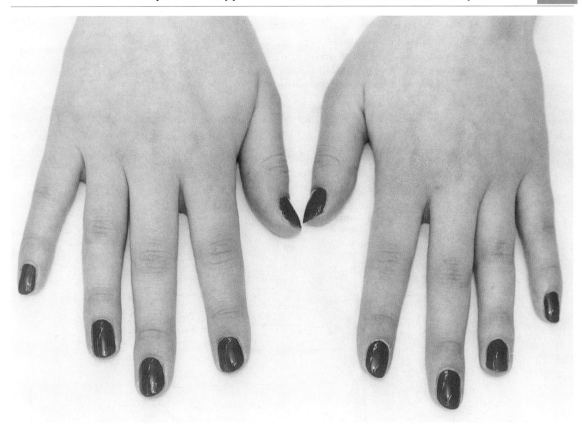

INTRODUCTION

The word 'Manicure' comes from the Latin *manus* – hand and *curo* – care. It involves treatment to improve the appearance of the hands and nails.

Manicuring is a popular service offered in beauty therapy clinics, hairdressing salons and nail salons. The treatment can be offered as part of other salon services e.g. hair styling, as part of a makeover in the beauty clinic or as preparation for nail extensions.

The purpose of manicure is to:
- recognise common nail disorders and disease
- provide a range of treatments to improve the hands and nails
- offer the client advice on nail care.

The manicurist has an ideal opportunity during the treatment to advise the client on other services available in the salon and to build a relationship with the client through conversation.

The manicure will include:
- filing and shaping the nails
- cuticle treatment
- hand massage

- nail varnish application or buffing
- special conditioning treatment.

THE STRUCTURE OF THE NAIL

The nail is made of layers of dead cells containing a protein called **keratin**, also found in skin and hair. The layers are held together by a substance called **lamellae**. The nail is divided into three main parts:

1. The **free-edge** – the part that protrudes over the fingertip
2. The **nail plate** – forming most of the visible portion of the nail
3. The **nail root** – the part of the nail buried into the skin.

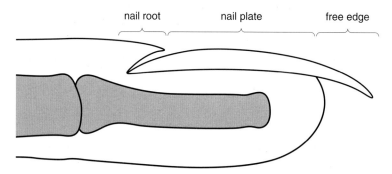

Figure 9.1 A cross section through the end of a finger and nail

The upper part of the nail forms the **nail fold** and the lower part forms the **matrix**. This is part of the germinating layer (stratum germinativum) of the epidermis and is the region from which the nail grows. The matrix receives the food and oxygen for growth from a network of blood vessels in the **nail bed**.

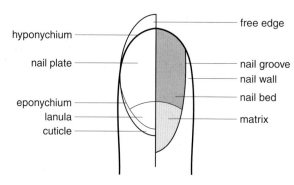

Figure 9.2 A cross section of nail in its bed

Part of nail	Description	Function
Free-edge	the part of the nail plate which protrudes over the fingertip, likened to the claws of an animal.	protects the fingertips from) physical harm (improves the appearance of the hands when manicured
Hyponychium	a layer of epidermis found under the free-edge	prevents bacteria and dirt from getting under the nail plate and infecting the nail bed
Nail plate	the main part of the nail, made up of layers of dead keratinised cells	protects the tips of the fingers and toes which have a network of sensory nerve endings
Lunula	also known as the half-moon, it is the visible portion of the matrix and appears pale due to a reduced blood supply	as the upper part of the matrix, it is part of the growing area for the nail – the nail plate and the nail bed are formed here
Cuticle	a layer of epidermis which overlaps the base of the nail plate	prevents bacteria and dirt from entering the nail fold
Eponychium	part of the cuticle at the base of the nail over the lunula which moves forward with the nail plate as it grows	protects the growing part of the nail
Matrix	lies beneath the nail fold – an injury to the matrix can cause deformity in the nail plate or the plate can be shed completely from the nail bed	the matrix has a rich blood supply which enables it to produce the nail plate and bed
Nail bed	this is the portion on which the nail plate rests, it has a plentiful blood supply when healthy and so gives the nail its pink colour	the blood supply provides the food and oxygen to the matrix and the ridges anchor the nail plate to prevent lifting, it also has a nerve supply making the nail bed sensitive to pain and pressure
Nail wall	the folds of skin running up the sides of the nail plate	forms the frame to the nail and provides protection from physical harm
Nail grooves	joined by the nail walls on either side of the nail plate	guides the nail to grow straight

Activity

Try to find the words listed below in the wordsearch.

Eponychium   Free-edge   Hyponychium   Nailplate   Matrix   Mantle   Lunula   Nail fold   Nail bed   Nail wall   Cuticle

Z	X	O	L	G	M	A	C	J	N	L	N	O	E	A	D
X	W	Y	J	K	A	D	F	G	A	M	P	R	T	S	U
C	C	A	B	W	T	X	Z	T	I	S	P	J	I	L	M
A	D	F	H	I	R	N	A	I	L	F	O	L	D	N	V
P	P	R	R	O	I	L	M	T	W	V	X	Z	W	I	L
N	B	N	D	E	X	I	R	T	A	M	A	N	T	L	E
A	F	A	G	H	E	J	D	K	L	U	A	L	O	U	R
S	T	I	R	P	U	E	C	E	L	I	G	H	V	N	W
Z	X	L	Y	W	B	O	D	D	L	H	A	C	B	U	J
E	O	P	A	L	U	P	S	G	T	C	U	R	V	L	W
X	U	L	I	Z	W	S	R	T	E	Y	I	V	H	A	I
L	M	A	O	N	P	O	J	B	D	N	E	T	C	Q	R
Z	N	T	Q	R	O	U	V	W	T	O	V	Q	U	B	C
D	L	E	U	V	Z	K	I	M	Q	P	X	M	R	C	Q
A	I	M	E	B	W	O	H	D	F	Y	V	H	T	V	X
F	G	O	T	E	P	O	N	Y	C	H	I	U	M	W	B

HEALTHY NAILS

Healthy nails appear firm but flexible, smooth and slightly pink in colour. The surrounding cuticle should be unbroken, flexible and should not be stuck down to the nail plate.

A healthy nail will grow approximately 3–4 mm per month and will grow faster in the summer, and in children and pregnant women. Children and pregnant women have higher levels of nutrients in the blood. In summer, due to the increase in temperature blood circulation is faster. Toenails grow more slowly than fingernails and are often thicker and harder.

To produce healthy nails the vitamins A, B complex and D are needed together with the minerals calcium and iron.

The effects of nail care treatment

Nail treatments such as buffing and massage benefit nail growth by increasing the blood supply to the nail bed. In doing so, more nutrients and oxygen are available for the cells to grow and divide. This means that the nails will grow more quickly and strongly.

The effects of illness

Systemic illness, in other words disease or illness affecting a system of the body, can influence the rate of growth and appearance of the nails, as well as the skin and hair. Poor health or poor diet can cause the nails to be brittle or very soft, flexible, pale, discoloured or blue in colour and the cuticles to be dry, split and hardened.

DAMAGE TO THE NAIL

Physical and chemical agents can cause nail damage.

Physical damage

Nail bed

A knock or blow that is hard enough to damage the nail bed will appear as a bruise under the nail. The blood vessels in the nail bed break allowing blood to flow out under the nail plate. After a little time the blood vessels mend, leaving some under the nail plate. This dries, sticks to the underside and grows up with the nail plate until it reaches the free-edge where it can be removed.

Matrix

Damage to the matrix can result in temporary loss of the nail or permanent damage to the nail plate. When the matrix is damaged by a severe knock or blow, some of the cells die. This results in a temporary halt in the production of the nail plate and nail bed. This can appear as a ridge in the nail or, if a lot of the matrix is damaged, the loss of the nail plate.

The dead cells need to be replaced and are made by the matrix itself. When fully healed, the matrix will begin to make the nail plate and nail bed again. If, however, the damage is severe enough, the matrix may not heal completely leaving scar tissue. This will appear as a permanent condition in the nail such as a vertical ridge or split.

Chemical damage

NAIL AND SKIN CONDITIONS WHICH CAN BENEFIT FROM TREATMENT

These are conditions which can be improved by nailcare treatments. In some cases they need special handling and this is noted where appropriate.

NAIL DISEASES AND DISORDERS

The presence of some conditions may contraindicate nailcare treatment. A therapist must be able to recognise conditions in order to make the decision as to whether a nailcare treatment can be

Condition	Cause	Appearance	Treatment
Corrugations	Vertical ridging can be hereditary or caused by damage of the matrix with age, indicating dryness. Horizontal ridging, if present on all nails, indicates a temporary pause in growth due to illness such as measles. If present on only one nail, the ridge may be caused by damage to the matrix.	Vertical or horizontal ridges or furrows within the nail plate.	If the ridging is mild, use a buffer with paste polish to buff the nails. Horizontal ridges grow out with the nail but avoid the use of coloured enamel as it is difficult to remove from the ridge. If ridging is severe treat the nails as fragile.
Bitten nails (onychophagy) See figure 9.3	Nervous or stressed induced habit.	The free-edge, nail plate and cuticle are bitten to leave the hyponychium exposed and the cuticle and surrounding skin ragged. Nail biting is the most common causes of deformed nails, due to the increased risk of infection.	Regular manicures help to overcome the habit. File the nails smooth to remove ragged edges, remove ragged cuticle, skin and hangnails with nippers to avoid temptation to bit. Give attention to the cuticles massaging with oil or cream.
Hangnails (agnail) See figure 9.4	Dryness, cutting off too much cuticle during manicure or the habit of chewing the cuticle.	Hard, dry pieces of nail or cuticle found in the nail groove or wall. If pulled, can result in torn tissue and subsequent infection.	Remove with cuticle nippers and suggest regular oil manicures which will prevent dryness.
Split nails (onychorrhexis)	Injury, filing too deeply into the nail wall, excessive use of solvents such as enamel remover, chemicals and alkalines, pressure on very long nails.	Horizontal or vertical splits in the free-edge, often at flesh level or below. When associated with dry hair and skin, this suggests a glandular disorder.	Perform oil manicures, use only the fine side of an emery board when filing, regular application of cuticle cream.

Condition	Cause	Appearance	Treatment
Brittle nails (fragilitas unguium)	Dehydration of the nail plate due to over exposure to alkaline, solvents, or immersion in water. Can also indicate an iron deficiency or anaemia.	Yellow, thick nails that break easily.	Avoid contact with chemicals and solvents, wear rubber gloves and use barrier creams. Regular use of cuticle cream especially at night.
Flaky nails See figure 9.5	Dryness caused by exposure to solvents and chemicals.	The layers of the nail plate separate at the free-edge.	Protect with gloves and barrier creams, regular use of nail strengtheners and cuticle cream, especially at night. File with the fine side of an emery board only and use enamel remover containing oil.
Blue nails See figure 9.6	Poor circulation due to cold, hereditary defect or heart disorder.	Nail plate appears blue instead of pink. May cause ridging of the nail plate.	Increase the circulation by exercise, massage and buffing.
White spots (leuconychia)	Mild injury to the base of the nail.	White spots within the nail plate. The injury causes the layers of the nail to separate.	They grow out with the nail plate. Avoid pressure on the cuticle during nailcare treatment. Use the fine side of an emery board when present in the free-edge.
Pterygium	It is either hereditary or can be caused by infrequent attention to the cuticle.	The cuticle is often dry, split and in excess, grows forward and sticks to the nail plate.	Careful use of the cuticle knife and nippers to remove the excess only. Oil manicures help prevent the regrowth from sticking back down to the nail and keeps the cuticle soft and supple.

Condition	Cause	Appearance	Treatment
Excess perspiration (hyperhydrosis)	Can be hereditary or caused by a stressful situation.	Hands or feet are damp and clammy. The feet can suffer from odour as they are confined within shoes.	Sweaty hands are difficult to treat, but a light dusting of ta c can help. Feet should be washed daily and anti-perspirant sprays or powders can be used. Socks or tights should always be worn and synthetic shoes should be avoided. Leather allows air to circulate around the feet. Special odour absorbing inner soles can also be used in footwear.
Hard skin (callous)	Thickening of the stratum corneum due to pressure and/. or overuse, formed to protect the affected area.	Dry, hard, inflexible overgrowth . over a bony prominence such as knuckles or joints.	Mild calluses may be removec by softening in warm water before the use of corn plane o· chemical hard skin remover. Severe calluses need referral to a chiropodist.

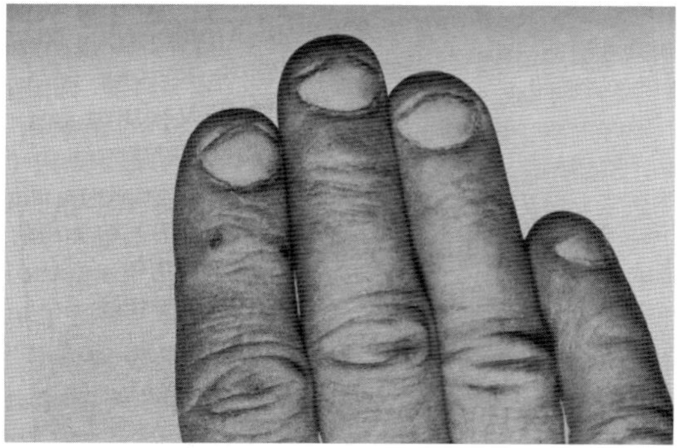

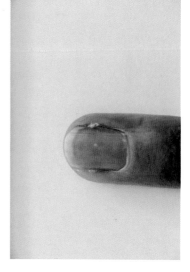

Figure 9.4 Hangnails

Figure 9.3 Bitten nails

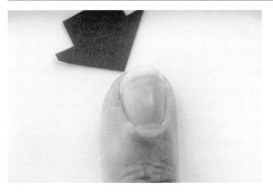

Figure 9.5 Flaky nails

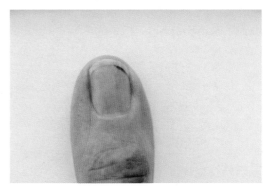

Figure 9.6 Blue nails

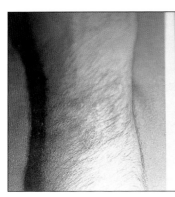
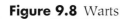

Figure 9.7 Ringworm

Figure 9.8 Warts

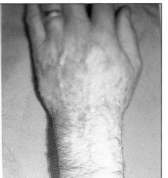

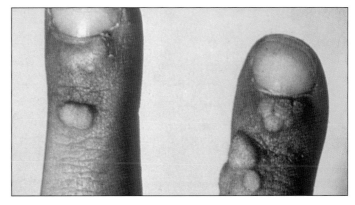

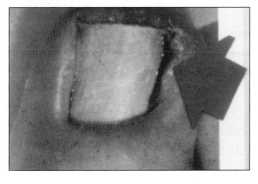

Figure 9.9 Whitlow

performed or not. The therapist must never make a diagnosis, but should refer the client to a specialist as appropriate. The signs of infection or inflammation are:

- redness
- swelling
- pain
- pus formation.

Contraindications

These can be divided into three types of condition:

1. Those that need medical referral.
2. Those that prevent treatment.
3. Those that restrict treatment.

1. Conditions requiring medical referral

Common diseases caused by the micro-organisms discussed in Unit 1. When referring a client it is important to do so without causing alarm or embarrassment.

Ringworm (Tinea)

Not a 'worm' as the name implies, but a fungal infection which can affect the nails and the skin. The disease is highly contagious and is often passed on by pets. Do not touch the area but tell the client to see a doctor as soon as possible.

Look out for:

- Yellow or white streaks and thickening of the nail plate. Sometimes the top layers of the nail will peel off. This is known as onychomycosis.
- Red, slightly raised patches of skin in the shape of a ring.
- On the feet, it appears as white, moist flaking or peeling between and around the bottom of the toes. Commonly called 'athlete's foot', it often spreads to the toenails.

Warts and verrucae

A contagious condition caused by a virus affecting the skin of the hands or feet (see Figure 9.8). Do not touch. If minor, they can be covered with a dressing and the treatment can be performed. If severe, the client should see a doctor. Look out for raised, horny lumps with black dots on the hands and horny lumps in an uneven shape which grow into the skin on the soles of the feet.

Whitlow (paronychia/onychia)

A contagious infection of the skin, cuticle or nail bed caused by bacteria entering through an opening in the skin or cuticle (see Figure 9.9). It can be caused by bad nailcare techniques but is usually associated with nail biting. Severe cases may need 'lancing' or a course of antibiotics, so advise the client to see a doctor. Look out for red painful swelling and the formation of pus.

2. Conditions preventing treatment
These conditions may need medical referral if severe. Mild cases can restrict treatment.

Eczema
An inflamed, red skin condition that is not contagious. It can be stress-related or the result of an allergy, for example to metals, chemicals, drugs, clothing or products such as nail enamels. If severe or with open sores, treatment would be contraindicated. When mild, however, treatment can go ahead, avoiding the area affected. Look out for redness, swelling, blisters, flaking, weeping and cracking of the skin. Eczema can give rise to changes in the nail such as ridging and pitting.

Dermatitis is a term used to describe any inflammation of the skin caused by an external irritant such as detergent.

Psoriasis
An inherited condition aggravated by stress, drugs, or infection. Commonly found on knees and elbows, it is not infectious so treatment can go ahead but with restrictions. Some nailcare treatments such as massage are thought to benefit the condition. However, if severe or open, cracked or infected, it is wise to refer the client to a doctor. Look out for:
- severe ridging or pits in the nail plate
- raised, red, silvery, scaly skin patches, circular or oval in shape with a definite outline.

Onycholysis
This term means the separation of the nail plate from the nail bed caused by systemic illness, injury, nail disease or infection, circulatory problems or as a reaction to drugs. It appears as a white area of the nail plate due to loss of blood supply. In severe cases, the nail plate may be shed completely or discoloration can be caused by the invasion of fungi or bacteria. If severe and of systemic or disease origin, the client should be referred to a doctor. Mild cases restrict treatment in that the affected finger should be omitted.

Bruised nail
Bruised nails are caused by injury to the nail bed with bleeding under the nail plate. There is dark purple, blue or black discoloration. Perform nail treatments with care, avoiding pressure. If severe, involving the loss of the nail plate, refer the client to a doctor. If mild, miss the finger out from the treatment. Cover with a dark coloured enamel if appropriate.

Chilblains
Caused by poor blood circulation and, therefore, common on fingers and toes. They are worse in cold weather. When severe, refer the client or delay treatment until the condition has improved. If mild, avoid the affected area. Look out for red, itchy swellings that become painful in the cold.

Ingrowing toe nails (onychocrytosis)

Can affect the fingers, but most common on the toes. The edges of the nail cut into the nail wall, which then can become infected by bacteria. The problem is caused by restrictive footwear, by clipping the corners of the nail too low at the nail wall or it can be a congenital defect. If inflammation or infection is present, the client should be referred to a doctor, if not the condition should be referred to a chiropodist and the nail omitted from the nailcare treatment.

3. Conditions restricting treatment

Corns

These are similar to calluses in that they are formed by an increase in pressure or over-use. A corn, however, develops a root-like structure that penetrates into the skin and when it presses on a nerve it causes pain. A client with a deep, developed corn needs referral to a chiropodist. Soft, new corns can be treated in the same way as calluses.

Bunions (hallus vulgus)

This is a condition where the big toe is forced towards and under the other toes due to pressure and friction from tight or pointed footwear. This causes the joint to swell and become inflamed causing pain. Another cause may be an inherited weakness in the arches of the foot. The therapist can assist with massage when the bunion is newly formed but in most cases the condition needs to be treated by a chiropodist or by referral to a doctor for surgery. During pedicure, take care with the area as pressure may be painful. Filing and cuticle work can be performed with care although enamelling may be difficult if the toe is severely affected.

Arthritis

There are two types of arthritis. Osteo-arthritis is the wear and tear of the joints and is more common in elderly clients. Rheumatoid arthritis is a disease that can affect a person at any age. Both involve painful joints, especially with movement or weight bearing. The conditions are usually treated with drugs and physiotherapy but, when under control, gentle massage can mobilise joints and eliminate fluid, reducing swelling. Such treatment should only be performed by a therapist with medical permission. The heat associated with paraffin wax treatments can give relief to painful joints.

Activity

Using the information you have been given, match the following descriptions with the conditions. Join the condition and the treatment with a line.

Hangnails	Lines or ridges in nail plate
Bruised nails	Ragged nail and/or nail cuticle
Corrugations	Hard, dry cuticle or nail
Brittle nails	Vertical or horizontal splits in the nail plate
Bitten nails	Yellow, thick nail which snaps easily
Split nails	Dark purple or black under the nail plate

Activity

Tick the box to show whether or not these nail and skin conditions should be referred to a doctor.

Condition	Needs to Refer	
	Yes	No
bruised nail		
split nails		
ringworm		
verrucae		
corrugations		
athlete's foot		
brittle nails		
whitlow		
warts		
hangnails		
bitten nails		
psoriasis		
chilblains		

BONES OF THE FOREARM, HAND, LOWER LEG AND FOOT

The forearm and hand

The **humerus** is a long bone which extends from the shoulder joint and forms the upper arm. The bone of the shoulder is called the **scapula**. The other end of the humerus forms a joint with the bones of the forearm. This is called the **elbow**. The long bones of the forearm are called the **ulna** and **radius**.

The ulna

The ulna is slightly larger than the radius and runs down the little finger side of the forearm. It forms the knobbly part of the elbow and its function is weight support and muscle attachment.

The radius

The radius runs down the thumb side of the forearm and is smaller than the ulna. This long bone is mainly concerned with muscle attachment. The radius and ulna form a joint at the elbow that allows the palm to turn forwards and backwards. At the other end, the radius and ulna form a series of joints with the bones of the wrist, known as the **carpals**.

The carpals

This is the group name given to the eight bones of the wrist. The bones are arranged into two rows of four. The uppermost row, the **scaphoid, lunate, triquetral** and **pisiform** form joints with the radius and ulna. The lower row, the **trapezium, trapezoid, capitate** and **hamate**, form a joint with the bones of the palm. The bones glide or slide over each other to allow a variety of movements.

The metacarpals

This is the name for the bones of the palm of the hand. There are five long bones in each hand, one relating to each of the digits.

The phalanges

This is the name given to the small bones making up the fingers and thumbs. There are 14 in each hand and these are arranged with three in each finger and two in the thumb.

The diagram opposite shows the relationship of these bones with each other and gives the names of each of the carpals.

The lower leg and foot

The long bone forming the thigh is called the **femur**. It extends from the hip to the knee. The function is one of support and muscle attachment. It forms a joint with the bones of the lower leg at the knee. These bones are called the **tibia** and **fibula**.

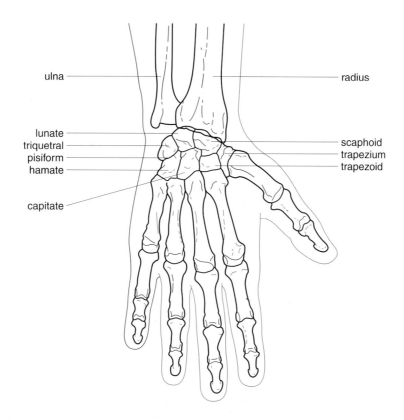

ulna

radius

lunate
triquetral
pisiform
hamate

scaphoid
trapezium
trapezoid

capitate

Figure 9.10 Bones of the hand

The tibia

The tibia is a long, strong bone situated towards the middle of the body and supports the body weight, as well as being used for muscle attachment. It forms a joint with the **talus** at the ankle.

The fibula

The fibula is a long slim bone situated towards the outer side of the lower leg. It is used mainly for muscle attachment. It forms a joint with the tibia near the knee and extends down to form joints with the ankle bones.

The patella

This is a flat bone situated at the knee joint commonly known as the **knee-cap**. It forms no joint with other bones because it is embedded in the strong tendon of the quadricep muscles in the front of the thigh.

The tarsals

The tarsals are seven bones which make up the ankle. They are larger than the carpals and are arranged differently to support the body weight and distribute it throughout the foot. The **talus** forms a joint with the tibia and fibula. The **calcaneum** performs an important function attaching the muscles of the calf in the lower leg to the foot, allowing powerful movements such as walking and running. The **cuboid** and **medial**, **intermediate** and **lateral cuneiform** form joints with the bones of the foot. The **navicular** lies to the inside of the talus and is used for muscle attachment and movement.

The metatarsals

These are five long bones making up the length of the foot. They form joints with the tarsals at one end and the bones of the toes at the other.

The phalanges

There are 14 phalanges in the toes arranged in a similar way to those of the hand. Two to the big toe and three in all the other digits, although those in the little toe are often fused together.

Below is a diagram showing the relationship and arrangement of these bones.

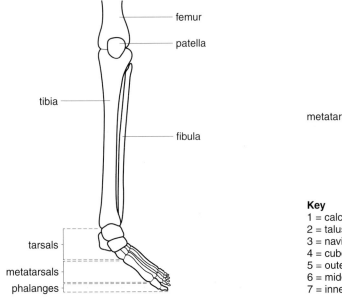

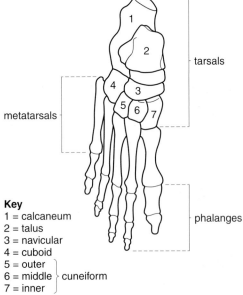

Key
1 = calcaneum
2 = talus
3 = navicular
4 = cuboid
5 = outer ⎫
6 = middle ⎬ cuneiform
7 = inner ⎭

Figure 9.11 a b Bones of the leg and foot

MUSCLES OF THE ARM AND LEG

Movement is brought about by the contraction of the muscles which are attached to the bones of the arm and leg across **synovial joints**. To reverse a particular movement another muscle must contract. For example, to bend the elbow, the biceps muscle contracts. To straighten the elbow, the triceps muscle contracts. The biceps and triceps are known as an **antagonistic** pair. Virtually all movements of the body are brought about in this way. The muscles listed below are antagonistic pairs. In cases where there is more than one muscle that brings about a movement, they are listed together.

Before you look at the list of muscles there is terminology that needs explaining.

Terminology
- Anterior = front
- Posterior = back
- Medial = the middle, towards the midline
- Dorsal = back
- Lateral = side
- Flexion = decreases the angle between two bones
- Extension = increases the angle between two bones
- Abduction = away from the midline
- Adduction = towards the midline
- Rotation = pivot about the joint
- Pronate = palm down
- Supinate = palm up
- Invert = towards the midline
- Evert = away from the midline
- Dorsiflex = toes toward the knee
- Plantarflex = pointed toes

Muscles of the arm
Biceps
- **Position** – found at the anterior aspect of the upper arm above the elbow. It is attached to the scapula bone at one end and the radius at the other.
- **Action** – flexes the elbow and supinates the hand and forearm.

Brachialis
- **Position** – attached to the humerus and ulna across the elbow.
- **Action** – flexes the elbow.

Triceps
- **Position** – found at the posterior aspect of the upper arm, it attaches to the scapula and humerus at one end and the ulna at the other.
- **Action** – extends the elbow.

Supinator

- **Position** – muscle attached to the lateral aspect of the lower humerus and the radius.
- **Action** – supinates the hand and forearm.

Pronators

- **Position** – muscle attached to the medial aspect of the lower humerus and the radius.
- **Action** – pronates the hand and forearm.

Flexors

- **Position** – muscle found at the medial aspect of the forearm attached to the lower humerus, radius and ulna at one end and the metacarpals and phalanges of the fingers at the other.
- **Action** – flex the wrist, fingers and thumbs.

Extensors

- **Position** – muscle found at the lateral aspect of the forearm attached to the lower humerus, radius and ulna at one end and the metacarpals and phalanges at the other.
- **Action** – extend the wrist, fingers and thumb.

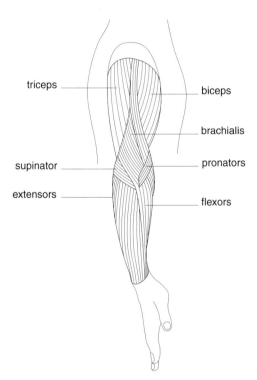

Figure 9.12 Muscles of the arm

Muscles of the hand

There are three muscle bulks in the hand which provide the strength needed for gripping actions.

Hypothenar eminence

- **Position** – in the palm of the hand below the little finger attached to the carpals and metacarpals and the phalanges of the little finger.
- **Action** – abducts, adducts and flexes the little finger.

Thenar eminence

- **Position** – found in the palm of the hand below the thumb. Attached to the carpals and metacarpals and the phalanges of the thumb.
- **Action** – abducts, adducts and flexes the thumb and draws it towards the palm.

Mid-palm group

- **Position** – centre of the palm below the middle three fingers. Attached to the carpals and metacarpals and phalanges of the middle three fingers.
- **Action** – abduct, adduct and flex the middle three fingers.

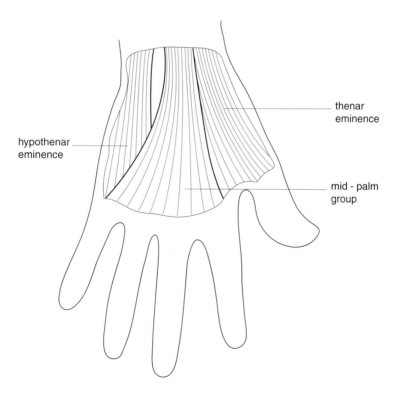

Figure 9.13 Muscles of the hand

Muscles of the thigh

There are many short, strong muscles present in the pelvic girdle that provide stability and cause movement of the hip. Due to the depth of these muscles they remain unaffected by massage and consequently are not listed here. Many muscles of the thigh and buttocks are listed by their group names rather than individually.

Quadriceps

- **Position** – a group consisting of four muscles found at the anterior aspect of the thigh attached to the pelvic girdle and the femur at one end and passing over the knee joint to the tibia bone at the other.
- **Action** – extend the knee and flex the hip.

Hamstrings

- **Position** – a group of three muscles at the posterior aspects of the thigh attached to pelvic girdle passing over the hip and back of knee to the tibia.
- **Action** – flex the knee and extend the hip.

Gluteus maximus

- **Position** – forms the buttocks. Attached to the pelvic girdle at one end and the posterior aspect of the femur at the other.
- **Action** – extends hip.

Adductors

- **Position** – a group of muscles positioned to the inside or medially of the thigh. Attached to the pelvic girdle at one end and the femur and tibia at the other.
- **Action** – to adduct and rotate the leg.

Abductors

- **Position** – a group of muscles including the **gluteus medius** and **minimus** found at the lateral aspect of the thigh and hip. Attached to the upper part of the pelvic girdle at one end and the upper aspect of the femur.
- **Action** – Abduct and rotate the leg.

Sartorius

- **Position** – attached to the pelvic girdle laterally, runs across the front of the thigh diagonally to the medial aspect of the tibia.
- **Action** – due to its unusual position, this muscle can flex both the hip and knee and abducts and rotates the leg.

Muscles of the lower leg and foot

Gastrocnemius

- **Position** – posterior aspect of lower leg, main muscle forming the calf. Attached to the lower part of the femur across the back of the knee and ankle to the calcaneum.
- **Action** – plantarflexes the ankle and flexes the knee.

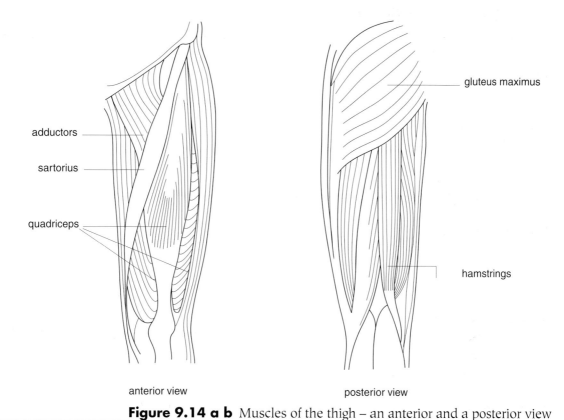

Figure 9.14 a b Muscles of the thigh – an anterior and a posterior view

Soleus

- **Position** – under the gastrocnemius in the calf, attached to the tibia and fibula at one end and across the ankle to the calcaneum at the other.
- **Action** – plantarflexes the ankle. Plantarflexion or pointing of the toes is an important action for propelling the body forward in walking and running.

Tibialis anterior

- **Position** – anterior aspect of the lower leg along the skin, attached to the tibia at one end and the medial cuneiform and first metatarsal at the other.
- **Action** – dorsiflexes the ankle and inverts the foot.

Tibialis posterior

- **Position** – posterior aspect very deep in the calf. Attached to the tibia and fibula at one end and the navicular bone on the other.
- **Action** – inverts the foot.

Peroneus

- **Position** – a group of three muscles found in the lateral and posterior aspect of the lower leg. They attach to the fibula and across the ankle to the underneath of the first and fifth metatarsal.

■ **Action** – evert the foot.

Flexors of the toes

■ **Position** – muscles deep in the posterior aspect of the lower leg attached to the tibia and fibula at one end and the phalanges of the toes at the other.
■ **Action** – flex toes and help plantarflex ankle.

Extensors of the toes

■ **Position** – muscle anterior and lateral aspects of the lower leg attached to the tibia and fibula and the phalanges of the toes.
■ **Action** – extend the toes and help dorsiflex the ankle.

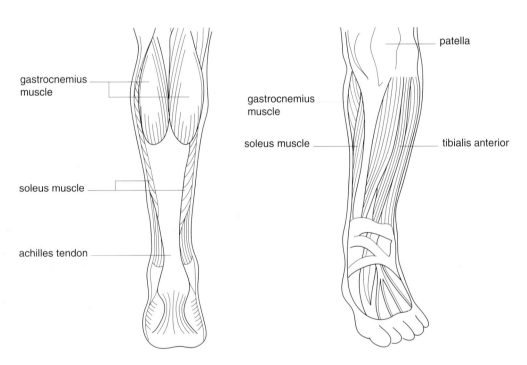

Figure 9.15 Muscles of the lower leg and foot

BLOOD SUPPLY TO THE ARM AND HAND

The blood supply to the arm begins with the **subclavian artery** which has branched off the **aorta**. The subclavian artery becomes the **axillary artery** and then the **brachial artery** which

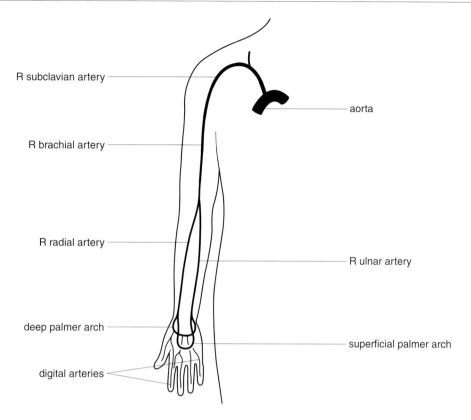

Figure 9.16 Arteries of arm and hand

runs down the inner aspect of the upper arm to about one centimetre below the elbow where it divides into the **radial** and **ulnar arteries**. The radial artery runs down the forearm next to the radius bone to the wrist where it nears the surface and can be felt as the **radial pulse**. It continues over the carpals to pass between the first and second metacarpal into the palm. The ulnar artery runs down the forearm next to the ulna bone, across the carpels into the palm of the hand. Together they form two arches in the hand, the **deep** and **superficial palmar arches**. From all these arteries branch others to supply blood to the structures of the upper arm, forearm, hand and fingers.

The venous return of blood from the hand begins with the **palmar arch** and **plexus** which is a network of capillaries present in the palm. Three veins carry the deoxygenated blood up the forearm: the **radial vein**, the **ulnar vein** and the **median vein**. The former two run parallel to the bones of the same name, the latter runs up the middle. Just above the elbow, the radial and ulnar veins join to become the **brachial vein**, and the median vein joins the **basilic vein** which originated just below the elbow along with the **cephalic vein**. As the veins continue over the elbow they link to form a network which eventually divides with the basilic vein joining the brachial vein which then becomes the **axillary vein**. The cephalic vein travels up the arm separately and becomes the **subclavian vein** in the upper chest.

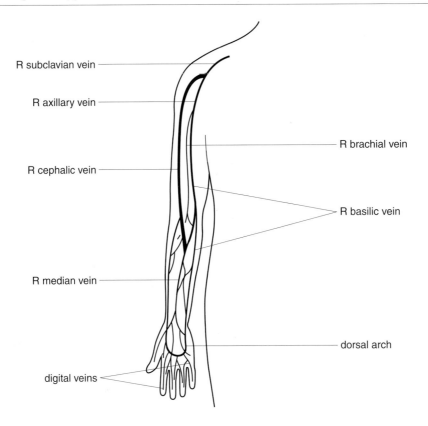

Figure 9.17 Veins of arm and hand

BLOOD SUPPLY TO THE LEG AND FOOT

The aorta travels down the length of the trunk to the lower abdomen where it divides into two arteries which supply either leg. The artery in the thigh is called the **femoral artery**, named after the bone of the thigh. At the knee the femoral artery becomes the **popliteal artery** which divides into two below the knee. One of these arteries runs down the front of the lower leg and is called the **anterior tibial artery**, while the other runs down the back and is known as the **posterior tibial artery**. This artery divides at the inside of the ankle becoming the **medial plantar artery** on the inside of the foot and the **plantar arch** on the sole of the foot. The anterior tibial artery becomes the **dorsalis pedis** on top of the foot.

There is a network of veins in the foot which become the **dorsal venous arch** on top of the foot. This travels the inside of the foot to the ankle where it becomes the **small saphenous vein**. It continues up the back of the whole leg to the thigh where it is known as the **great saphenous vein**. Two small veins called the **anterior tibial veins** travel up the front of the lower leg while two veins, the **posterior tibial veins** run up the back. These four veins converge just below the knee to become the **popliteal vein** at the back of the knee and then eventually the **femoral**

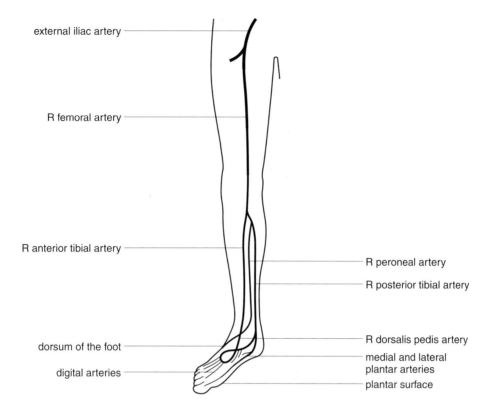

external iliac artery

R femoral artery

R anterior tibial artery

R peroneal artery

R posterior tibial artery

R dorsalis pedis artery

dorsum of the foot

medial and lateral
plantar arteries

digital arteries

plantar surface

Figure 9.18 Arteries of the leg and feet

vein in the thigh. The great saphenous vein and the femoral vein join at the groin and return to the heart.

LYMPH DRAINAGE OF THE ARM AND LEG

The lymph drainage from the arms and legs travels in one direction following the venous flow to the heart. The major lymph nodes are found in the crease of the elbow and in the armpit for the arm, and at the back of knee and front groin in the leg.

Lymph drainage works against gravity. Tissue fluid can collect in the feet and ankles causing swelling. This is more likely if the person has a job that involves them standing still for long periods of time.

THE NERVES OF THE ARM AND LEG

General information about the nervous system can be found in Unit 6. The 31 pairs of spinal nerves are numbered according to the section of the spinal column from which they arise:

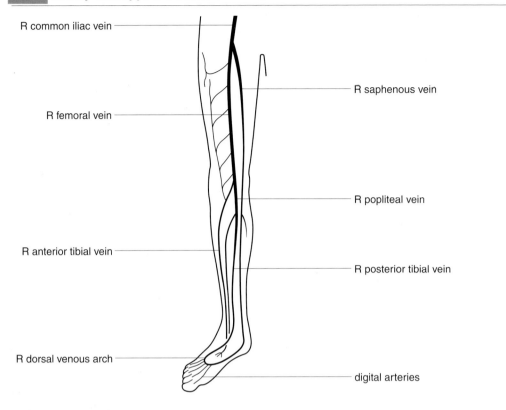

R common iliac vein

R saphenous vein

R femoral vein

R popliteal vein

R anterior tibial vein

R posterior tibial vein

R dorsal venous arch

digital arteries

Figure 9.19 Veins of the leg and feet

- 8 pairs of cervical nerves (neck region)
- 12 pairs of thoracic nerves (chest region)
- 5 pairs of lumbar nerves (lower back region)
- 5 pairs of sacral nerves (bottom region)
- 1 pair of coccygeal nerves (tail region)

The fifth to eighth cervical nerves (C) serve the arm and the second to fifth lumbar (L) and first to second sacral (S) nerves, the leg. Due to the size of the muscles of the limbs, a large muscle may be served by more than one nerve. It is easier, therefore, to list the nerves according to the muscles they serve.

The arm		The leg	
Muscle	**Nerve**	**Muscle**	**Nerve**
Deltoid	C5 and 6	Gluteus Maximus	L5, S1 and 2
Biceps	C5 and 6	Quadriceps	L3, 4 and 5 and S1
Brachialis	C5 and 6	Hamstrings	L4 and 5 and S1 and 2
Triceps	C7	Adductors	L2, 3 and 4
Flexors	C6, 7 and 8	Abductors	L4 and 5
		Sartorius	L2 and 3
Extensors	C6 and 7	Gastrocremius	L5 and S1
Supinator	C5 and 6	Soleus	L5, S1 and 2
Pronators	C6 and 8	Anterior Tibialis	L2, 3 and 4
		Extensors of toes	L5 and S1
		Flexors of toes	L5, S1 and 2
		Peroneus	L5 and S1
		Posterior Tibialis	L4 and 5

NOTE! For a Key Skills Task for this unit see page 133.

Element 9.1

Assess clients and prepare a treatment plan

NOTE! For more information on this element see page 153.

CLIENT CONSULTATION AND TREATMENT PLANNING FOR MANICURE

Client consultation is a very important part of the service offered to a client. It should be carried out prior to every treatment whether the client comes for treatment regularly or for a one–off visit.

A client's health and circumstances can change between visits to the salon so it is important to go through the consultation process every time. It may be that you need to check progress against the treatment plan.

Details of treatment planning can be found in Unit 5.

Assessing the clients hands and nails for manicure

Firstly clean the client's hands with cotton wool and surgical spirit. This will give you the opportunity to make a quick assessment of the overall condition.

Assessing the client for treatment involves:
- **Look** – looking at the hands
- **Touch** – touching the skin
- **Question** – questioning the client.

Look and touch

1. **The palms and backs of both hands**. Check for rough, dry patches of skin, any cuts or broken skin, sore areas where rings are worn and the colour of the skin, whether red and chapped or pigmentation marks. The age of the client will affect the texture of the skin and disease such as arthritis may be apparent.

2. **The cuticles**. The condition of the cuticle of the nails will immediately indicate whether the client cares for her hand and has regular manicures. Over grown, torn and dry cuticles will require extra work during the manicure and home care advice to the client.

   Hangnail is a common condition where the cuticle becomes attached to the nail plate and it tears as the nail grows. Infection may then result. Biting the nails and cuticle also leads to thick and torn cuticle.

3. **The nails**. Inspect each nail for:
   - **shape** – there are many different shaped nails. A distorted shape may be the result of nail damage.
   - **colour** – slightly pink colour is an indication of healthy nails. Discoloured nails may be the result of smoking or may be caused by the client's work, as in the case of the hairdresser who works with products which colour the hair. (As hair and nails are of a similar composition, that is made from the protein keratin, the nails will take on the colour in a similar way to the hair.
   - **strength** – nails will vary in thickness, flexibility and strength. This is normally an hereditary factor although illness, disease and certain drugs can severely affect the condition of the nails. Flaking and splits in the nail should be noted.

It is essential that you can recognise nail disorders and disease to establish contraindications. Refer to page 239–247 for details.

Question

Discussion with the client at this stage is a very important part of the consultation. If there are any conditions of the hands or nails which are contraindications and prevent you continuing with treatment, this must be handled in a very sensitive manner. An explanation of the condition and why it prevents you from continuing must be given to the client. This will usually be because there is infection present which could be passed on to other clients or therapists. It may be appropriate to explain to the client how the condition could spread and infect others in the home or work place.

Gentle questioning will enable you to establish the lifestyle, habits and occupation of the client, all of which will have an effect on the condition of the clients hands and nails. You may be able to establish the cause of a condition by asking an open question:

- Tell me how do you look after your hands and nails at home?
- What kind of work do you do with your hands?

By talking to the client you will be able to identify the client's needs and expectations. You will be required to advise her on what the treatment entails, what the end result will be and whether you can meet her expectations. It is important that you discuss the cost of the manicure, especially if you have agreed to include a special treatment which will take extra time.

The questioning phase of the client assessment will allow you to build a rapport with the client and help her to relax, making the treatment more enjoyable.

All of the details that you discover through looking, touching and questioning should be included in the treatment plan or record card.

Activity

1 Look closely at your hands. Write down what you see. Following the look, touch, question routine. Now repeat the exercise on a colleague.

2 Observe as many different nail shapes as you can by looking at friends, family, and in magazines.

Contraindications to manicure

1. Infection in the area of the hands and nails recognised by the presence of **redness, swelling, pain** and **puss**.
2. Infectious nail disease.
3. Open cuts and abrasions.
4. Allergic reaction to manicure products, the symptoms being: **itching, swelling, redness, raised blisters**.

Activity

A teenage girl appears at reception enquiring about treatment for nail biting. She reluctantly displays her hands to the manicurist, which shows severely bitten nails. She is a nervous and shy person. She explains that she is taking school exams at the moment but will finish school in two weeks time.

1   Write a short paragraph on how you think this client is feeling as she discusses her hands and nails with the manicurist, how the manicurist should handle the client and what advice should be given.

2   Write out a treatment plan for this client to include both salon and home care.

Activity

Describe four adverse nail conditions, including clearly labelled diagrams of the nail and the nail bed.
Briefly describe for each condition:

1   salon treatment.

2   home care advice.

Element 9.2

Prepare the work areas and client for manicure and pedicure treatment

PREPARING THE WORK AREA FOR A MANICURE

As a manicurist you may be called upon to treat a client in a whole range of different situations: whilst the client is having other treatment in the beauty therapy salon or in a hairdressing salon where it will be necessary to move to the client. This will require portable equipment, either a movable manicure station which is a stool with a small table and drawers to hold products and implements or a light weight stool with products and implements carried in a basket.

Wherever you work, it is essential that:

■ seating for the client and manicurist is comfortable ; you should not be in a slouching position as this can cause back problems over a period of time and will certainly cause fatigue

■ there is good lighting – it may be necessary to have a magnifying lamp or an angle poise lamp to hand

■ there is adequate ventilation – when working with solvents it is essential that fresh air circulates freely (this applies particularly when using artificial nail systems).

■ manicure implements are clean, sterilised and arranged in a neat and organised manner with everything to hand

■ hot and cold water with liquid soap is available for washing your hands before and after treatment, for soaking the clients nails to soften the cuticle and to remove preparations from the nails during treatment

■ there are plenty of clean towels available.

Client care and preparation

Before examining your client's hands ensure that you have washed your hands thoroughly using a medicated hand wash to minimise the risk of cross infection.

Ensure that your client is seated comfortably. Ask her to remove rings, bracelets or watches which may hinder the manicure treatment, particularly the massage where hand cream could become lodged between the settings of the jewellery. The client's jewellery should be kept near the client, on the trolley in a small bowl.

The client's cuffs or sleeves need to be turned back and protected with tissue during massaging to avoid clothing coming into contact with manicure products which may stain.

Before carrying out a manicure treatment the client must be consulted to establish **contraindications** to the treatment (see page 244).

Preparation and hygiene procedures

Preparation and hygiene procedures are an essential part of **all** salon treatments. Manicure implements are small items which can be cleaned and sterilised quite easily and some are disposable. The trolley, whether a specialised manicure trolley with drawers and compartments for storing tools and products or an equipment trolley, must be wiped over with disinfectant. Sterilised and clean tools need to be set out in an orderly way which allows the manicurist to have them close at hand whilst working. A manicure basket may be used by the mobile therapist.

Refer to Unit 1 for details on general health, safety and hygiene procedure.

PRODUCTS, IMPLEMENTS AND EQUIPMENT

Implements used in manicure

- **Nail scissors** – small curved blades for reducing the length of the nails.
- **Cuticle knife** – small, flat blade used to remove cuticle attached to the nail plate.
- **Cuticle nippers** – small scissor like implement with a spring action to allow small movements, used to remove excessive, torn or damaged cuticle.

> **NOTE!** All these items can be washed in hot soapy water and sterilised using an autoclave. They can be stored in an ultra violet cabinet after sterilising. During the manicure small implements should be placed in disinfectant on the trolley.

- **Buffer** – an implement which has a surface covered with chamois leather. Applied to the surface of the nail plate to create a shine using brisk rubbing (friction).

> **NOTE!** The chamois leather cover can be wiped over after use with a damp cloth. The leather covers need changing regularly.

- **Hoof stick** – orange wood or plastic handle with a rubber end shaped like a hoof, used to gently push back the cuticle from the nail plate.
- **Nail brush** – used to remove all manicure products before the application of nail varnish, may also be required to clean dirty nails.
- **Orange stick** – wooden implement with a slanted end and a pointed end which should be tipped with cotton wool before use. The orange stick has a number of uses: pushing back softened cuticle with cotton wool tipped end soaked in cuticle remover, to clean under the nails with pointed end tipped with cotton wool and to remove small amounts of preparations from their pots.
- **Spatula** – used to dispense products from plots (maybe made from plastic material which can easily be washed or wood which can be disposed of after use).

> **NOTE!** These items of small equipment can be washed in hot soapy water and placed in the ultra violet cabinet for storage. The orange stick, spatula and hoof stick should be placed in disinfectant during the manicure.

- **Emery board** – has a dark side which is coarse and used when nails are to be shortened in length or for filing very strong nails. The light side is fine and used for shaping and smoothing the nails. The emery board should be flexible and 12–15 cm long to allow for good technique during filing of the nails.

> **NOTE!** Emery boards are made of fibrous board and therefore cannot be washed. They should be offered to the client for use at home or thrown away after use.

Products used in manicure

- **Varnish remover** – a solvent which removes nail varnish. **Amyl acetate** or **acetone** are the main ingredients in varnish remover with a small amount of oil added to help counteract the drying effect of the solvent on the nail plate.

- **Cuticle massage cream** – an emollient used to soften and nourish the cuticles. **Lanolin** or **mineral oils** are the main ingredients. Cuticle oil may be used in the same way.

- **Cuticle remover** – an alkaline substance which softens the keratin in the skin, allowing the cuticle to be lifted from the nail plate and excess to be removed using cuticle nippers. **Potassium hydroxide** is the main ingredient which is caustic and very drying if not removed thoroughly after use. Cuticle remover also has a mild bleaching effect and can help to remove stains from the nails.

- **Buffing paste** – a mild abrasive substance which, when combined with the friction action of the buffer, gives the surface of the nail plate a shine. **Pumice**, **silica** or **stannic oxide** (jeweller's paste) is the main ingredient. Buffing may help increase the circulation to the nail bed and smooth ridges in the nail.

- **Hand cream/lotion** – an emollient which softens and nourishes the skin and assists in the application of massage. **Lanolin**, **glycerol** or **vegetable oils** are used to make an oil-in-water emulsion. Other ingredients include perfume and colour.

- **Nail varnish: base coat, top coat and coloured varnish** – a plastic film which is applied to the nail plate. **Nitro cellulose** and a solvent such as **amyl acetate** are the main ingredients of all nail polish, with various pigments added to give colour or guanine from fish scales to give a pearlised effect. Good quality nail varnish lasts longer, has a good range of colours, has a good consistency for smooth application and dries quickly and evenly.

- **Base coat** – provides a smooth base for the application of coloured varnish, protects the nails from staining which can be caused by colour pigment, minimise ridges or irregularities in the nail plate and prolongs the life or varnish by helping to prevent chipping and peeling.

- **Top coat** – is used to give extra gloss to cream varnish and to help the varnish last longer by providing a hard surface, protecting the varnish from chipping. Top coat is not required for crystalline varnish as it can dull the finish.

- **Nail polish thinners** – a solvent used to thin down nail varnish which has become thick. **Ethyl acetate** is the active ingredient and should be used very sparingly otherwise the varnish will not harden. Nail varnish remover should not be used for thinning varnish as the oil it contains will prevent the varnish from drying.

- **Nail strengthener** – a product which hardens the keratin in the nail plate. **Formaldehyde** is the active ingredient in these products. Nail strengthener may also be an acrylic substance which provides a hard plastic coating to reinforce the nail.

- **Nail white pencil** – a pencil which is dipped in water before applying to the underside of the free edge. This whitens stained nails. **Titanium dioxide** is the main ingredient.

- **Quick dry spray** – the cooling effect can speed up the drying process. A **solvent** aerosol spray which evaporates quickly is the basis of this product, although polish which is allowed to dry naturally is longer lasting.

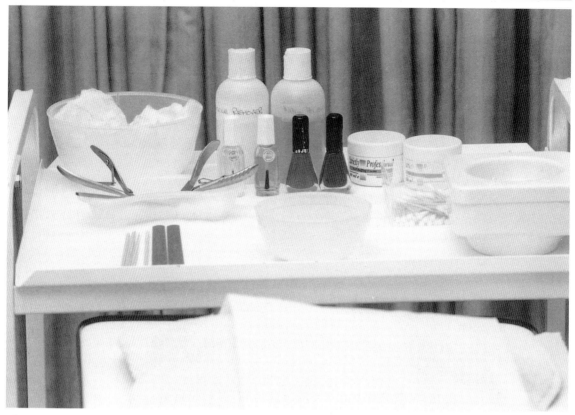

Figure 9.20 Layout of the manicure trolley

Activity

1 Familiarise yourself with the products used in your salon by reading the labels and manufacturer's instructions, checking the colour, consistency and smell.

2 Make a list of the products needed for a manicure.

3 Visit a department store or chemist shop and look at the range and cost of products and tools available to your clients.

General items of equipment and materials

As well as specialist items of equipment and products, you will need some more general equipment and materials which include.

- **Surgical spirit** – for cleansing the client's hands prior to examination and for disinfecting implements and surfaces.
- **Jar of sanitising fluid** – to hold manicure implements during treatment. This may be disinfectant or sterilising fluid.

- **Cotton wool** – for wiping over the hands when soaked in surgical spirit, for removing nail polish when soaked in polish remover and for tipping the orange stick before use.
- **Tissues** – for wrapping sterilised implements before use, for covering the towelling cushion during polish application to protect the towel.
- **Towels** – for drying client's hands during the manicure. A towel should be placed on your lap during the manicure for drying your hands.
- **Finger bowl** – filled with hot water and a few drops of medicated liquid soap for soaking the client's hands. (The water will have cooled sufficiently by the time the client needs to immerse her hand.)
- **Small receptacle** – for holding your client's jewellery safely whilst carrying out the manicure.
- **Waste bin** – for immediate disposal of waste materials. A small pedal bin is ideal.

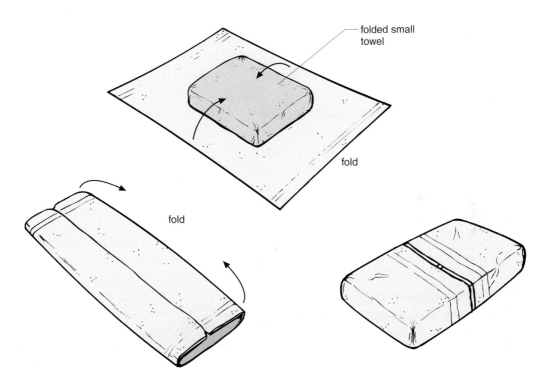

folded small towel

fold

fold

Figure 9.21 Forming a manicure cushion with towels

HYGIENE PROCEDURES AND CARE OF SMALL IMPLEMENTS AND MANICURE PRODUCTS

Small implements

Always buy good quality stainless steel manicure tools such as the cuticle knife and nippers, so that they can be sterilised without damaging them. Make sure blades are sharp, particularly the cuticle nippers to avoid tearing the cuticle. Ensure that the hinge moves easily on the nippers to allow for the correct technique to be used.

All small tools must be sterilised after use whether by autoclave or chemical sterilising fluid as appropriate, (refer to Unit 1 for sterilising methods). The items should be dried and stored either in an ultra violet cabinet or placed in a tool roll.

Products

Many manicure products contain solvents and must, therefore, be handled and stored carefully. The COSHH risk assessment for your salon will identify hazards when using these products. (For details of COSHH regulations refer to Unit 1).

It is important that tops are secure on bottles to avoid evaporation of varnish remover and varnish thinners.

Particular attention is needed when caring for nail varnish. Your clients will want to choose from a wide range of varnish colours. Varnish should be of excellent quality to ensure a long lasting finish and good colours.

The necks of the bottles should be wiped after use to ensure that the top fits securely. When the solvent is allowed to evaporate from the varnish, it becomes thick and impossible to apply to the nails. Varnish will require thorough shaking before use to ensure a smooth well mixed colour. Small beads are placed in some bottles to ensure thorough mixing. Slight separation may occur in cream varnishes, leaving a white deposit or sometimes dark layers form at the top of the bottle.

Coloured varnish needs to be stored upright, away from direct sunlight to avoid fading of colour pigments and thickening of the varnish due to changes in temperature.

Activity

Tick the boxes as you prepare for your first manicure.

Is the manicure area warm and tidy ☐

Do you have clean towels available ☐

Implements

cuticle nippers ☐

cuticle knife ☐

emery board ☐

buffer ☐

orange stick ☐

hoof stick ☐

spatula ☐

Materials and equipment

manicure trolley/table ☐

stool ☐

water bowl ☐

waste bin ☐

cotton wool ☐

tissues ☐

manicure cushion ☐

jar of sterilising fluid or disinfectant ☐

bowl for clients jewellery ☐

Products

varnish remover ☐

cuticle massage cream ☐

nail scissors ☐

buffing paste ☐

hand cream ☐

base coat ☐

coloured varnishes ☐

top coat ☐

nail strengthener ☐

nail white pencil ☐

quick dry spray ☐

french manicure products ☐

SELF ASSESSMENT TEST

1. What is the main reason for using buffing paste when buffing?
    a) to stimulate nail growth
    b) to condition the nails
    c) to improve the colour of the nails
    d) to give the nails shine.
2. Nitrocellulose is an ingredient found in:
    a) cuticle remover
    b) buffing paste
    c) nail varnish
    d) hand cream.
3. When shaping the nail the emery board should be used:
    a) with a sawing action across the top of the free edge
    b) in one direction towards the centre of the free edge
    c) across the surface of the nail plate
    d) by pulling back the nail wall and filing the free edge to a point.

4. Which product contains a solvent?
   a) hand cream
   b) buffing paste
   c) cuticle remover
   d) varnish remover.

5. Which is the correct way to hold a cuticle knife, to ensure that the blade and not the point is used is?
   a) in an upright position between the thumb and first finger
   b) to hold like a pen
   c) flat in the palm of the hand with the thumb and first finger guiding the implement
   d) between the thumb and middle finger.

6. Hot water is essential during the manicure:
   a) to soak the client's nails and cuticles
   b) to wash the towels
   c) to clean the manicure implements
   d) to wipe up any spillages.

Element 9.3

Improve the appearance of nails and skin using manicure and pedicure techniques

WORK METHOD FOR MANICURE

Having cleansed the client's hands by wiping with surgical spirit, checked for contraindications and discussed the treatment plan with the client. You can begin the manicure.

Quick reference guide for manicure

The following is a quick reference guide to the work method for manicure. Each stage is explained in more detail later in this unit.

1. Remove nail varnish from the nails of both hands.
2. File the nails of the left hand (buffing can be done at this stage without buffing paste).
3. Apply cuticle massage cream.
4. Soak left hand in the bowl of warm soapy water.
5. Repeat steps 3 and 4 on the right hand.
6. Dry left hand thoroughly.
7. Soak the right hand.
8. Treat the cuticles on the left hand by applying cuticle remover and pushing back the cuticle using a cotton wool tipped orange stick and a hoof stick.
9. Remove excess cuticle using the cuticle knife and cuticle nippers.
10. Use the nail brush to rinse off cuticle remover and any loose cuticle. Dry thoroughly.
11. Repeat steps 6–10 on the right hand.
12. Massage both hands.
13. Remove grease from the nail plate on each hand using cotton and varnish remover.
14. Apply nail varnish. Base coat (once), coloured nail varnish (twice) and top coat (once). If the client does not want nail varnish buff to a shine.
15. Allow varnish to dry completely. Offer the client home care advice.

PROCEDURE
Removing nail varnish

1. Apply nail varnish remover to a pad of cotton wool. Hold between your first two fingers to avoid remover smudging varnish on your own nails.
2. Press the pad firmly on to each nail and hold allowing the solvent to dissolve the cellulose coating on the nail.
3. Slide off the nail in one movement, from the base of the nail to the free edge, to prevent the colour spreading over the finger.
4. It is some times necessary to repeat with fresh cotton wool or to apply remover to a cotton wool tipped orange stick and remove colour from around the cuticle.

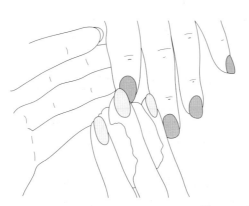

Figure 9.22 Removing nail enamel

5. Ensure there are no traces of old varnish as this will spoil the benefits of treatment and final appearance of the nails.

6. Remember to place the top on the bottle of remover to prevent the solvent evaporating.

Shaping the nails

This is an important stage in the manicure. You must discuss the shaping of the nails with the client. They may have very strong views. There are a number of factors which must be taken into consideration at this stage:

■ Natural shape and length of the nails – are they equal in length and shape?

■ Condition and strength of the nails – are the nails brittle, dry, thin?

■ Client's occupation.

■ Shape of the hands and fingers.

■ **Oval** – the ideal shape as it provides strength to the free edge.

■ **Square** – a square shape is popular, particularly for long nails and nail extensions.

■ **Pointed** – pointed nails require shaping down the nail wall which causes weakness to the free edge. Splits low down in the nail plate can result.

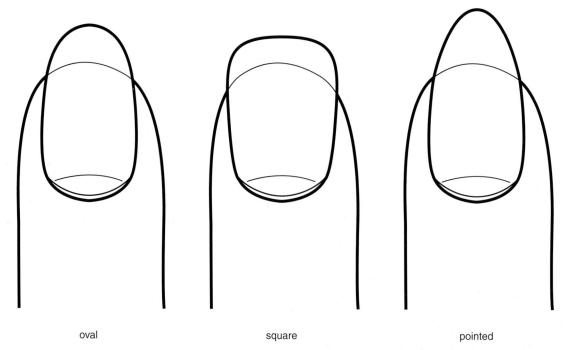

oval   square   pointed

Figure 9.23 The effects of different nail shapes

> **NOTE!** Therapists do not usually wear nail varnish as it can mask dirt under their nails. Manicurists, however, may have varnished nails.

Shortening the nails

It may be necessary to shorten excessively long nails. This is best carried out using sharp, curved nail scissors followed by filing. The nail should be supported whilst cutting the free edge. Very hard brittle nails may require soaking first. The nail should be cut straight across leaving it slightly longer than the finished shape to allow for filing.

Filing

Good quality emery boards should always be used. They should be flexible and 12–15 cm in length to allow long sweeping movements when filing. The emery board will have different degrees of coarseness on either side, indicated by the colour. The dark side is coarse and used for reducing the length of strong nails. The finer side is light in colour and used for shaping and smoothing the nails. The emery board should be held with the thumb on the side not being used and four fingers on the other side.

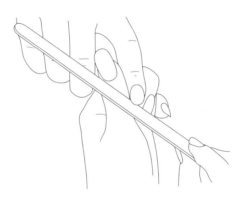

Figure 9.24 Filing nails

Nails must be filed in one direction, from the side to the centre of the nail tip, making an oval shaped movement. Long, swift, rhythmical strokes should be used. Sawing movements backwards and forwards can damage the nail, particularly if soft and delicate. Filing into the corners of the nail by pulling back the nail wall will weaken the nails and reduce the support to the free edge. This can lead to split and breaking of the nail.

Bevelling is used after shaping to remove any fragments left after filing and to smooth the edge of the nail. The fine side is used to file under the free edge at 45 degrees.

Cuticle treatment

The aim of treatment is to reduce dryness and overgrown, torn or thick cuticles leaving the skin around the nail neat, soft and pliable.

Cuticle work is an important stage in the manicure. The treatment required will depend on the condition of the client's hands and nails. It may take several manicures to treat poor cuticles. This should be indicated in the treatment plan.

Cuticle massage cream is applied first. A small amount is dispensed from the pot using an orange stick and applied to each nail. The cream is massaged into the nail and surrounding skin. The emollient makes the cuticles pliable and the massage increases circulation to the tips of the fingers.

Soaking the fingers in hot soapy water will soften the skin and clean the nails.

Cuticle remover and using implements is the next stage of cuticle treatment. One of the major problems with untreated cuticles is that the skin adheres to the nail plate and becomes torn causing hangnails. Cuticle remover and the use of special implements to remove cuticle from the nail plate and trim excess cuticle from around the nail is advised.

After soaking the hands are dried and cuticle remover applied all around the cuticle and under the free edge. Cuticle remover is slightly caustic and breaks down the keratin in the skin allowing the cuticle to be loosened. It may also remove stains from the nail plate.

A cotton wool tipped **orange stick** is used to push back the cuticle. A rolling movement is used starting half way up the nail plate and rolling down to the base of the nail, gently pushing back the cuticle.

The **hoof stick** with its flexible rubber hoof-shaped end, is designed to continue the lifting of cuticle from the nail plate. Use flat circular movements, working downwards to the base of the nail plate.

The **cuticle knife** should be held flat in the palm of the hand, not upright between the thumb and first finger or like a pencil. The flat position ensures that the length of the blade is used to gently 'scrape' any cuticle sticking to the nail plate, rather than using the point of the blade which could damage the matrix.

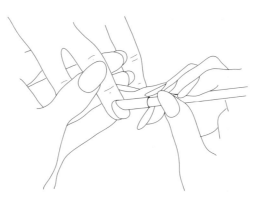

Figure 9.25 Pushing back cuticles

The blade is stroked in one direction and must be moistened throughout by dipping into the manicure bowl. This prevents scratching the nail plate.

Cleansing under the free edge to remove dirt and dead skin is carried out using a cotton wool tipped orange stick, taking care not to dig into the nail bed.

The **cuticle nippers** are used to cut away excess cuticle which has been lifted from the nail plate during treatment or to cut off torn cuticle. Some clients require careful cuticle work at this stage, due to overgrown or damaged cuticles, often caused by the client biting the nails and surrounding skin or lack of care to hands and nails resulting in dryness and damage.

Hangnail may be treated but special care must be taken not to pull at the skin, causing discomfort to the client.

Excessive forward growing cuticle (**pterygium**) can be improved with very careful use of cuticle nippers. Cuticle nippers must be handled very carefully to avoid tearing the cuticle and causing bleeding which could lead to infection.

The aim is to remove the cuticle in one piece so that there are no rough edges. This requires the correct holding of the nippers. They should be held in the palm of the hand with the spring between the handles moving smoothly. The nipper blades are then used in a 'nibbling' action in a curved movement around the base of the nail.

Pulling the cuticle as a result of poor technique or blunt blades will cause tearing and possibly bleeding. Trimming the cuticles too closely will weaken the protection they give to the nail and increase the risk of infection.

It is not always necessary to use the cuticle nippers. For example clients who have regular manicures and a good home care routine may not accumulate a great deal of cuticle.

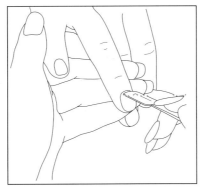

Figure 9.26 Using a cuticle knife

The **nail brush** is used next. Dipping the treated nails into the water in the manicure bowl, the brush is used from the cuticle to the free edge. This gets rid of the dead skin removed during this stage of the manicure and, most importantly, flushes away the cuticle remover which is slightly caustic and, if left on the nails, would be very drying.

Inspect the nails and cuticles

When cuticle work is completed on both hands it is important to evaluate the treatment so far. Visual checks should include:

- Are the nails an even shape?
- Does the free edge of the nails need bevelling to remove any layers or snags left after filing?
- Do the nails require any repair?
- Are the cuticles pushed back exposing as much lanula as possible?

Any minor shaping or correcting rough or torn cuticle should be done at this stage.

You should gain the clients approval and refer to the treatment plan. Any future treatment to improve the nails and surrounding skin should be discussed and recorded in the treatments plan.

Hand massage

Hand massage can be the most enjoyable part of the manicure for the client. You must allow sufficient time to ensure that the massage is not rushed and that the full benefits of the massage can experienced.

The benefits of hand massage are to:
- relax the client
- increase the blood and lymphatic flow to the hands and fingers
- improve mobility in the joints
- spread the hand cream or lotion
- nourish and smooth the surface of the skin by helping the skin to absorb the hand cream
- remove loose skin cells.

Massage of the hand uses:
- **Effleurage** – stroking movements using the palm of the hand or the tips of the fingers. These are flowing movements using very little pressure to spread the hand cream. Effleurage is applied in an upward movement, towards the heart and should start and end the routine.
- **Petrissage** – kneading movements, which are deeper and more stimulating. Petrissage increases lymphatic and blood flow and can aid the removal of loose skin cells.
- **Rotations** – circular movements applied to the joints to aid mobility.

Where possible the client should remove long sleeved items of clothing or roll sleeves up to the elbow to prevent hand cream from soiling clothing. The client may wish to have massage to the lower arm and hand, in which case short sleeves are essential. Otherwise the massage is applied to the wrist and hand only.

Massage routine
The area to be massaged can be divided into:
- the forearm and elbow
- the wrist
- the palm and back of the hand
- the digits (fingers)

If your routine follows a set pattern it will make it easier for you to remember and ensure a thorough massage.

Quick reference guide for hand massage
This is a quick reference guide to help you whilst you are practicing. The full procedure follows.

1. Apply sufficient handcream.
2. Effleurage from fingers to the elbow 3–4 times.
3. Petrissage (thumb kneading) to the forearm wrist to elbow 3 times.
4. Thumb knead the top of wrist (carpels).
5. Criss-cross thumb movements (friction) to the under side of wrist.
6. Rotate wrist 3 times in each direction.

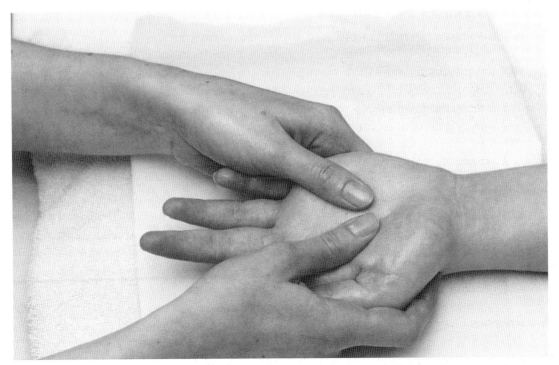

Figure 9.27 Hand massage

7. Flex wrist 2–3 times.
8. Thumb knead the back of the hand.
9. Thumb knead the palm.
10. Thumb knead the joints of the finger.
11. Rotate fingers 3 times in each direction.
12. Finger 'snapping'.
13. Effleurage to finish.

The forearm

1. Take sufficient hand cream from the container using a spatula or pour lotion directly into your hands. Take care not to apply too much lotion as it becomes messy and your hands will not massage effectively if the skin is too slippery. It is also unnecessarily extravagant and wasteful.
2. Effleurage from the fingers to the elbow with a small amount of pressure to spread the cream evenly. Support the client's hand and mould your other hand around the upper surface of the arm as you move up to the elbow. Return moving down the underside of the arm. It should not be necessary for you to alternate your hands, use which ever is most natural and comfortable to you. Repeat 3–4 times.
3. Petrissage (thumb kneading) to the forearm using the thumb of one hand in circular movements, whilst supporting the client's arm with the other hand. Slide back down to the wrist and repeat.

The wrist

1. Thumb knead the wrist using small circular movements, as if you were feeling for all the intricate little bones of the wrist.
2. Apply rapid thumb movements (friction) in a criss-cross action to the inside of the wrist. This stimulates the main artery (radial) leading to the hand.
3. Rotate the wrist by placing the client's elbow on the manicure cushion and whilst supporting the forearm grip the fingers and rotate in one direction and then the other. Repeat 6 times in each direction.
4. Flex the wrist by placing the client's elbow on the manicure cushion and whilst supporting the forearm interlock your fingers with the clients and push the hand back slowly and firmly. Repeat 2–3 times.

Palm and back of the hand

1. Thumb knead the back of the hand from the knuckles to the wrist using both thumbs in circular movements.
2. Thumb knead the palm by turning the hand over and applying deep circular movements with both thumbs to the fleshy part of the palm.

The fingers

1. Thumb knead the joints of the fingers and thumb.
2. Rotate fingers by supporting the hand and holding each finger individually, rotate first in one direction 3 times and then in the other.

3. Finger 'snapping' – use in the first two fingers of your hand to twist and pull the finger from the knuckle to the finger tip, as if pulling blood through the vessels to the very tip of the finger.

To complete the massage

The final movement in the massage routine is to effleurage the hand and forearm 5–6 times, finishing with your hand slowly working to the tips of the client's fingers, placing them on the manicure cushion. The client's hand can be wrapped in a towel to keep it warm whilst repeating the massage routine on the other hand.

Effleurage can be used to link movements together or to warm up an area which has not been worked on for some time and may be getting cold.

Buffing

Buffing may be incorporated in the manicure at one of two stages in the routine:

1. After filing, without using buffing paste, to increase the circulation to the nail or with buffing paste to begin smoothing the surface of the nail plate. Nails with small ridges may benefit from buffing with paste as it is slightly abrasive. Deep ridges or damage to the nail plate will not be reduced by buffing.
2. After hand massage as an alternative to nail varnish:
   ■ for male clients
   ■ clients who want a natural shine to their nails
   ■ for those in occupations where varnish would not be appropriate for hygiene reasons: nurses, those working with food.

Buffing method

1. A very small amount of buffing paste is taken from the container using an orange stick. Care should be taken not to use too much paste or to spread it onto the cuticle, as it is difficult to remove.
2. Place a small dot of paste on the centre of each nail plate of the hand being treated.

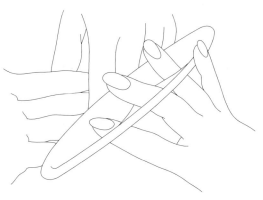

Figure 9.28 Nail buffing

3. Spread the paste towards the free edge with a ball of the thumb before using the buffer.

4. Hold the buffer between the first two fingers although this may depend on the style of the buffer. Holding the buffer correctly ensures that a light movement can be used therefore avoiding thumping the nail.

5. Stroke the buffer fairly quickly **in one direction only** from the cuticle to the free edge 15–20 times for each nail or until you have created a shine. Ensure that buffing paste is not spread onto the surrounding skin.

Choosing nail varnish

You would normally discuss the colour type of nail varnish with the client during the consultation. The client may have definite views or rely on you to advise. The choice of colour should be recorded on the record card.

Points to be considered when choosing varnish are:

■ The age and colour of the skin – older hands which are uneven in colour and have red and blue tones do not suit orange and peach colours.

■ Bright colours draw attention to the hands and require the nails to be an even length and shape.

■ Dark nail varnish will draw attention to the nails and make small nails look even smaller.

■ Pearlised varnish shows up any imperfections in the nail plate.

■ A special occasion may require matching of the varnish to an outfit or other make-up colouring.

Nail varnish application

The final stage of the manicure is the application of nail varnish. Ensure that you have allowed sufficient time when planning the treatment for careful application.

1. Place a tissue over the manicure cushion to avoid spoiling the towels.

2. Ask the client to replace jewellery to avoid smudging the nail varnish at the end of treatment. Ensure that the nails are free from grease and manicure preparations by wiping over with nail varnish remover on cotton wool. Make sure there are no cotton wool fibres left on the nails.

3. It may be appropriate to ask the client to pay for the treatment at this stage so there is no risk of damaging the finished application.

4. Apply a base coat first, followed by two coats of coloured varnish and then a top coat. Pearlised crystalline and frosted varnish do not require top coat, so a third coat of colour may be applied.

5. To avoid risk of smudging the varnish during the application it is a good idea for the right handed manicurist to start with the little finger of the client's left hand and work towards the thumb, repeating on the right hand. (The left handed manicurist should reverse the procedure.)

6. The way in which the clients finger is supported is important to prevent catching the nails during the application.

The colours and style of application of varnish will depend on fashion and to some extent the length and shape of the nails:

- the whole of the nail plate can be varnished
- the lanula can be left unvarnished
- the nail plate can be varnished leaving a gap at the sides, to give an illusion of length which is particularly useful on broad thumb nails
- the nail plate can be varnished natural pink, with free edge varnished white (**French manicure**).

Allergic reaction to nail varnish

Formaldehyde resin is thought to be the cause of allergy to nail varnish. Itchiness and inflammation, followed by dry flaking skin is likely to occur around the eyes or areas where the nails come into contact with the skin such as the face and neck.

Removing excess varnish

Varnishing the nails is very skilled work and requires a great deal of practice. The most experienced manicurists sometimes make mistakes and too much varnish on the brush can lead to flooding of the cuticle. This can be rectified by using a cotton wool tipped orange stick dipped in varnish remover to carefully work around the cuticle taking off any varnish. This method should only be used when occasional mistakes are made during application. You must aim to apply polish without catching the surrounding skin.

Drying

It is essential that the varnish is completely dry before the client leaves the salon. If possible, each coat should be allowed to dry before the next one is applied. Thick and poor quality varnishes or over thinned varnish may not dry in the time available, so should be avoided. The client may request revarnishing if the varnish smudges after a reasonable amount of time. Quick-drying aerosols can speed up drying time by the rapid evaporation of the spray on the nails. A fine film of oil is left behind which reduces the tackiness of newly varnished nails.

Repairing a smudge

It can be extremely annoying if the client or the manicurist catches the nails before the varnish is dry. It the nail is badly smudged, then it is advisable to remove the polish from the nail and reapply starting with base coat. Sometimes a minor smudge can be dealt with by applying varnish remover to the nail. This must be done carefully by applying varnish remover to the tip of your finger and smoothing over the smudged nail in one direction towards the free edge.

This may be repeated taking care not to flood the nail with remover.

If successful the nail should be left to dry and a further coat of coloured varnish applied if necessary.

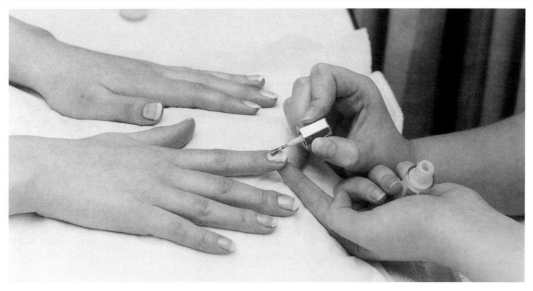

Figure 9.29 Applying nail varnish

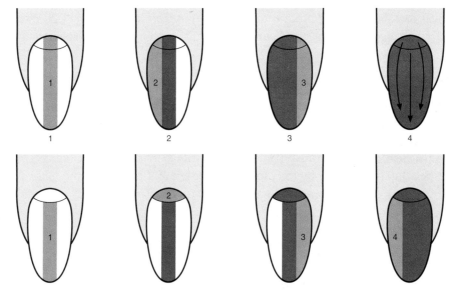

Figure 9.30 Different varnish applications

Activity

Select a dark coloured varnish and ask three friends or colleagues with different nail shapes and lengths to act as models. For example:

■ short square shaped nails

■ long oval shaped nails

■ misshaped nails

Begin by wiping over the nails with varnish remover and apply a base coat. Do not choose old thick varnishes just because you are practising. Apply two coats. Do not use an orange stick to remove polish from the cuticle.

Evaluate your varnish application in each case using the following checklist and add a comment on the suitability of the dark colour for each of the models.

Varnish application checklist	Yes	No
Was the varnish a good consistency?	☐	☐
Did you start with the finger and work towards the thumb?	☐	☐
Did you use the minimum number of strokes to apply the varnish?	☐	☐
Was the varnish smooth on the nail?	☐	☐
Did the varnish cover the nail plate evenly?	☐	☐
Was there any varnish on the cuticle or surrounding skin?	☐	☐
Were any of the nails smudged?	☐	☐

After care advice

Offering the client after care advice is an important part of salon service.

You can use the opportunity to:
- advise on home care
- recommend further treatment
- retail cosmetics.

Advise the client to:
- wear protective gloves when doing gardening, housework and washing up as detergents and chemicals will dry the skin and nails
- dry the hands thoroughly after washing and apply hand cream
- protect the hands in cold weather by wearing warm gloves
- use hand cream and cuticle cream just before going to bed
- not to use finger nails to open lids
- protect weak and brittle nails with nail strengthener
- always use an emery board for filing the nails, not a metal file as they create heat by friction and dry out the nail plate
- buff the nails as this will improve circulation to the nail bed and give the nails a natural shine
- ensure a good diet – supply of calcium, iron and vitamin A are necessary for nail health.

PEDICURE

Care of the feet

In general, people do not look after their feet. Women in particular will follow fashion trends in foot wear at the expense of comfort and correct fitting shoes. This can lead to long term foot disorders such as bunions and calluses, as well as poor posture.

Choosing the correct shoes for every day wear, particularly for work, is important. For example the beauty therapist, who stands for long hours in a very warm environment, should choose shoes which support the foot. A good fit is necessary so that the toes are not cramped and heels not chafed causing blisters and hard skin.

A low heel rather than a flat shoe gives support to the arch of the foot. Equally, very high heels are extremely tiring if worn for long periods of time. They tend to change the natural posture by throwing the weight forward.

The purpose of pedicure is to:
- improve the appearance of the feet and nails
- relax tired and aching feet
- reduce hard skin on the feet
- offer advice on care of the feet and referral as necessary to a chiropodist.

The pedicure will include:
- shaping the nails
- cuticle treatment
- removal of hard skin
- foot massage
- nail varnish application as required.

> **NOTE!** much of the routine for manicure applies to pedicure.
> The major differences are:
> - the positioning of the client and therapist for treatment
> - the treatment of hard skin and the implements and products used
> - foot massage routine.

Contraindications to pedicure
- infectious conditions – clients may be unaware of conditions of the feet which require referral to a doctor or chiropodist (eg verrucae, athlete's foot)
- open wounds such as burst blisters, cuts or abrasions.

(See page 239 for details of nail disorders, which apply to feet as well as hands.)

Preparation and hygiene procedures for pedicure
All general hygiene procedures for salon treatments apply, as do the routine hygiene procedures for manicure relating to implements, equipment and the work area.
(Refer to pages 22–25 for details)

Client preparation
Soaking the client's feet prior to thorough examination and treatment is essential. A quick visual check of both feet is required and you should question the client regarding any foot problems.

1. Prepare a foot bowl with warm water and antiseptic liquid soap.
2. Place both feet in the water for 3–5 minutes. This will help relax the client, as well as freshen the feet prior to treatment.
3. It is a good idea at this stage to dry the feet with disposable paper towels in case, after closer examination, infectious foot disease is present.

Clients are often unaware of conditions such as athlete's foot and you may not be able to see it without close examination between the toes. This can be carried out discretely whilst drying the feet. The client can be advised and referred to a chiropodist or doctor. The treatment should be cancelled until the condition has cleared. The foot bowl will require disinfecting and you must wash your hands very thoroughly.

Products, implements and equipment
Pedicure treatment will require the same products and implements as for manicure with the following additions:
- foot bowl
- toe nail clippers
- cuticle trimmer
- callous file or corn rasp for removing hard skin
- exfoliating cream or hard skin remover
- toe separators
- (a buffer is not required).

Procedure for pedicure
The basic manicure routine is followed throughout, except where extra treatment is required to deal with foot specific conditions such as hard and dry skin and, thickened nails. These are discussed later in this unit.

Quick reference guide for pedicure
1. Soak both feet in warm soapy water.
2. Dry both feet with disposable paper and inspect the feet closely.
3. Remove nail varnish.
4. Replenish the water in the foot bath to ensure that it is warm.
5. Cut nails on the left foot with curved scissors or nail clippers.
6. File.
7. Apply cuticle massage cream.
8. Soak.
9. Repeat steps 5–8 on the other foot.
10. Dry the left foot thoroughly.
11. Soak the right foot (check with the client that the water is still warm).
12. Treat the cuticles on the left foot by applying cuticle remover and pushing back the cuticle using the cotton wool tipped orange stick.
13. Remove excess cuticle with the cuticle knife and cuticle nippers.

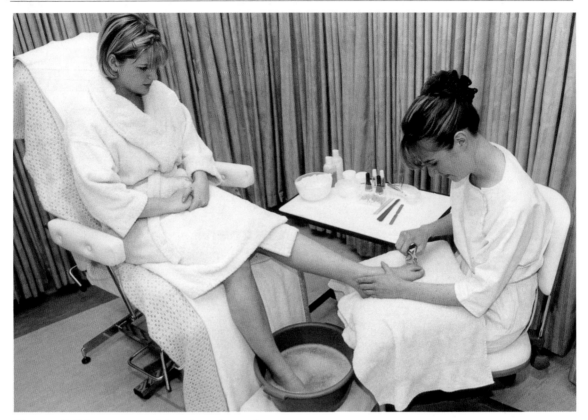

Figure 9.31 Position of the client for pedicure

14. Use a callous file or rasp if required to remove the build up of hard skin usually on the pads of the foot and heel.
15. Apply hard skin remover to the sole of the foot, heels and tops of the toes as required. Using the heel of the hand apply with vigorous rubbing to help exfoliate the hard skin.
16. Rinse off the cuticle remover, hard skin remover and exfoliated skin in the foot bath using a wad of cotton wool.
17. Dry the left foot and wrap in a dry towel to keep warm.
18. Repeat stages 12–17 on the right foot.
19. Massage both feet (and lower leg as required).
20. Remove grease from the nail plate on each foot with varnish remover on a pad of cotton wool.
21. Use toe separators or tissues twisted between the toes to separate the toes and prevent the varnish smudging.
22. Apply varnish. Base coat (once), coloured varnish (twice) and top coat (once).
23. Allow varnish to dry completely. This is absolutely essential before replacing tights/stockings and shoes.
24. Give home care advice to client.

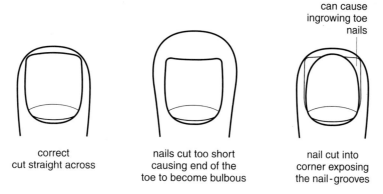

correct
cut straight across

nails cut too short
causing end of the
toe to become bulbous

can cause
ingrowing toe
nails

nail cut into
corner exposing
the nail-grooves

Figure 9.32 Toe nails cut correctly and incorrectly

Cutting the toe nails

Toe nails should be cut straight across to avoid ingrowing toe nails. After soaking the feet to soften the nails, the nail clippers or sharp scissors can be used, followed by filing with the course side of an emery board.

Pressure from wearing shoes can cause the nails to thicken, particularly the big toe nails. Thickened toe nails are particularly common in older clients. It may be necessary to refer the client to a chiropodist for nails to be cut.

The nails protect the ends of the toes and should not be cut too short as this will cause discomfort and pressure on the ends of the toes.

Cuticle work

The cuticles on the toes are often quite thick and overgrown unless the client cares for her feet and has regular pedicures. The cuticles can be treated in the same way as in a manicure, but extra time will be needed for using the cuticle nippers or cuticle trimmer to cut excess cuticle from around the nails. The cuticle trimmer should only be used on hard raised cuticle. It is a small V shaped implement. The V has a sharp cutting edge with trims excess cuticle as it is passed around the base of the nail.

Removing hard skin

Hard skin develops on the feet as a form of protection in those areas which receive the greatest pressure and rubbing. The balls of the feet and heels are commonly affected. You should remove or smooth only unsightly dry skin to improve the appearance of the feet. It is the job of the chiropodist to deal with excessive hard skin including calluses and corns.

There are a range of implements which can be used for treating hard skin. The callus file and corn rasp are metal files used to lift dead hard skin from the foot using a quick filing movement.

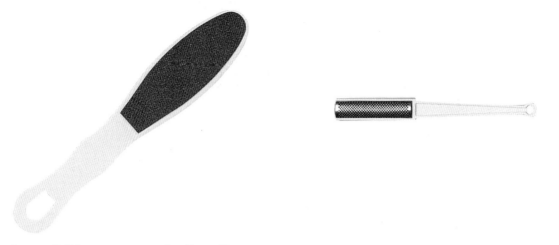

Figure 9.33 Corn rasp and callous file

FOOT MASSAGE

Foot massage is very relaxing for the client. It is important that the client is positioned comfortably to avoid strain as pressure is applied during the massage. Refer to page 292 for the benefits of massage and massage movements.

It is usual to massage the feet and lower leg, but if the client is wearing trousers she may wish to have just the feet and ankles treated. Remember to protect clothing from the lotion by using tissues.

Remember to follow a sequence as for hand massage dividing the area to be massaged into the:

■ lower leg
■ ankle
■ top and sole of the foot
■ toes.

Quick reference guide for foot massage

1. Apply sufficient hand cream.
2. Effleurage from foot to the knee 6 times.
3. Petrissage (thumb kneading) the front of the leg.
4. Petrissage the calf (palmar kneading).
5. Thumb kneading round the ankle bone.
6. Thumb kneading to the Achilles tendon.
7. Palmar kneading over the medial arch.
8. Thumb kneading underneath the foot and toes.
9. Hacking to the sole of the foot.

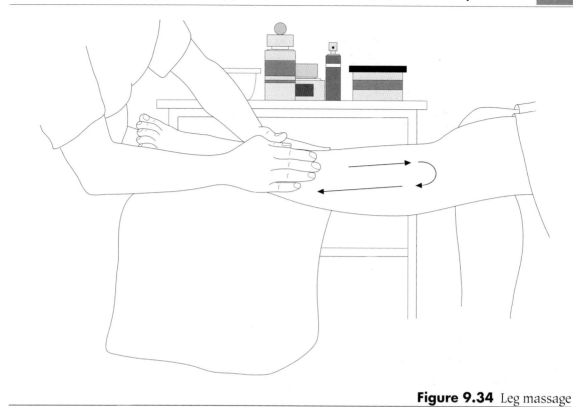

Figure 9.34 Leg massage

10. Deep stroking of the foot.
11. Whipping of the toes.
12. Toe snatching.
13. Effleurage to the leg and foot 6 times.

Nail varnish application

The procedure for varnish application is very similar to manicure, except the nails, apart from the big toe nail, are often very small making application more tedious.

Toes do not span naturally like fingers, so toe separators are required to keep them apart whilst the varnish is drying. Toe separators made from foam can be obtained from beauty suppliers but, as they cannot be sterilised easily, it is more appropriate to use folded tissues which can be disposed of after treatment. Cotton wool may be used but the fibres may get onto the nails and spoil the finished varnish application.

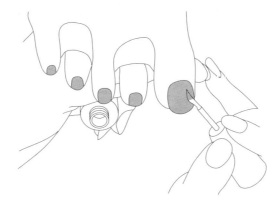

Figure 9.35 Applying varnish to toes

After care advice

Offering advice to your clients after the pedicure will help them look after their feet between visits. It is also an opportunity to recommend retail products such as foot powders, sprays, foot baths and hard skin remover.

After care advice will differ for each client depending on the condition of their feet. It may include the following:

■ wash feet daily (more often if suffering from excessively sweaty feet and in hot weather)
■ make sure feet are thoroughly dry after washing especially between the toes
■ change socks or tights daily
■ allow the air to circulate around the feet by going barefoot whenever it is comfortable and safe to do so
■ buy good quality shoes that fit properly (changing shoes with different heels can help with tired feet)
■ wearing very high heels over long periods of time should be avoided as they cause tired sore feet and poor posture
■ avoid wearing synthetic shoes such as trainers over long periods of time as they cause the feet to sweat
■ any infection or serious conditions of the feet must be referred to a doctor or chiropodist (regular visits to a chiropodist may be necessary for some clients with on going foot problems).

Evaluation of treatment

It is essential at the end of any treatment to evaluate the treatment against the treatment plan.

■ Have you met the client expectations? Are they satisfied with the pedicure? Have you done what you set out to do in your treatment plan? This could be special attention to the cuticle or hard skin removal, for example.
■ Was the pedicure carried out in a commercially acceptable time? A pedicure will take

longer then a manicure because of the time needed to treat the cuticles and hard skin. A client who cares for her feet and has regular pedicures will require 30–35 minutes for treatment. If the feet require extra attention 45–55 minutes will be needed. The time you expect to take should be discussed with the client as part of the treatment plan.

■ Was the pedicure of professional quality? You must aim to provide careful and accurate treatment in the best possible time to be commercially viable. Following your evaluation of the pedicure was it the best you could do or are there things which require improvements and more practice?

Activity

Using the check list on page 287 evaluate your pedicure treatment.
Evidence of your performance can be judged by:
■ the client's comments, enter verbal or written comments in your diary or log
■ colleagues in the work place, who work with you and observe you, ask them to provide a written witness testimony
■ your teacher or assessor who will mark your assessment book.

MANICURE FOR A MALE CLIENT

It is necessary to adapt the routine of the manicure to meet the needs of male clients. Less time is required for varnish application and shaping the nails and more time may be spent on cuticle work and hand massage.

1. File nails to a shorter length and a gentle round or square shape.
2. Use unperfumed hand cream for the hand massage.
3. Use deeper movements in the massage and increase the time for massage.
4. Buff the nails with buffing paste to create a natural shine, rather than using varnish. Some clients may wish to have a coat of clear varnish.

REVARNISH

Regular manicure clients may on occasions request that their nails are varnished without a full manicure. It may be that the client needs to change her nail colour between manicures to match an outfit or that she dislikes the colour applied. Whatever the reason, a revarnish must only be carried out on perfectly manicured nails to ensure that a professional finish can be achieved.

Revarnish routine

1. Cleanse the clients hand with surgical spirit in the normal way.
2. Briefly check the shape of the nails and file if necessary.

3. All traces of varnish must be removed on the left hand and fingers placed in the finger bowl to soak. This will remove all traces of varnish remover and cleanse the nails.
4. Remove the varnish from the other hand and place it in the manicure bowl, having removed the left hand.
5. Thoroughly dry the hand and check the cuticles. Remove any obvious bits of cuticle.
6. Apply hand cream and do a short massage routine to the hands.
7. Repeat on the other hand.
8. Wipe over the nails with varnish remover soaked in cotton wool.
9. Apply nail varnish in the usual way.

NAIL REPAIR

No method of nail repair will stand up to heavy daily work with the hands. As a temporary measure for a special occasion there are various methods of repairing fragile, split or flaking nails.

Causes of splits in the nail

A split may be in the free edge of the nail or below the free edge and may be due to:

- nails being too long and catching on clothing or catching when doing jobs without wearing gloves
- nails which are filed to a point are prone to splitting because there is less protection from the nail wall
- chewing or over trimming the cuticle so there is insufficient protection to the nail.

Causes of flaking/fragile nails

The nail is made up of layers of flat dead kerentinised cells. Sometimes these layers separate at the free edge and peel back. This may be due to:

- an hereditary condition – your client will tell you that she has never been able to grow her nails long without this happening.
- the diet
- illness can weaken the nails – may not be seen for several months
- using strong chemicals or immersing the hands constantly in water will weaken the nails.

Nail strengthening

Products are available to help prevent nails from splitting. Nail strengthening fluid applied to the free edge on a regular basis will harden the nails. These products contain formaldehyde and should be used with care following the manufacturer's instructions. Nail strengthening varnish is usually clear and can be used as a base coat. It provides extra coats of cellulose to the nail, forming a protective layer.

Nail repair products

Nail mending uses fibrous tissue and a fast drying adhesive or nitrocellulose. Nail repair glue or cement is also available.

Method of repair using mending tissue

The problem should be assessed during the client consultation and will be part of the treatment plan. Nail repair takes extra time and if you are planning improvement in the nails over a number of treatments this needs to be recorded. Nail repair is usually incorporated in the manicure during the application of the base coat. This method can be used as necessary between manicures but the nail must be free from varnish or hand cream.

1. Wipe over the nail with varnish remover.
2. Tear a small piece of fibrous tissue to the size of the split. (The tissue must be torn not cut to ensure that the edges are uneven. This allows the tissue to be blended onto the nail disguising the repair.)
3. The nail repair adhesive is applied to the nail plate including under the free edge and then to both sides of the tissue.
4. The tissue is placed over the split allowing about a third to extend beyond the free edge. This is then tucked under the free edge using an orange stick which has been dipped in varnish remover.
5. The tissue is smoothed onto the nail using the orange stick which must remain moistened with varnish remover. Smooth out any air bubbles blending the tissue as close to the nail as possible. This can be achieved with a little varnish remover applied to the pad of the thumb and carefully smoothing over the nail.
6. Turn the client's hand over and smooth the tissue under the free edge. Take care not to move the tissue and disturb the blending on the nail plate.
7. Apply a further layer of adhesive to the whole of the nail plate and allow to dry completely.
8. Coloured nail varnish can be applied as required.

Broken, split and flaking nails can be remedied by the application of **nail extensions**. Many salons offer this service and you may wish to refer your client to a nail technician for specialist advice.

1. free edge

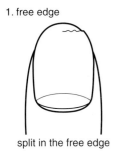 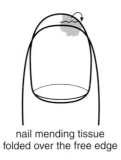

split in the free edge

nail mending tissue
folded over the free edge

2. below flesh line

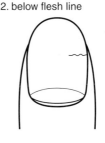 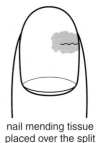

nail mending tissue
placed over the split
on the nail plate

Figure 9.36 Nail repair

Element 9.4

Improve the condition of nails and adjacent skin

HEAT TREATMENTS AND SKIN CONDITIONERS FOR THE HANDS AND NAILS

The therapist must make the most of opportunities for offering extra treatments to the client. This not only increases takings, but helps to keep the interest of the client as well as improving her appearance. There are a number of treatments which can add to the enjoyment of a manicure and which also help to improve the condition of the client's hands and nails.

Treatments used by the beauty therapist on other parts of the body, for example moisturising masks and exfoliating treatments, can be adapted for use on the hands and feet. The use of heat in conjunction with nourishing creams, oils or waxes can also be very beneficial. The heat required to increase the effectiveness and pleasure for the client can be supplied by:

- heating the material before application, as for paraffin wax or warm oil treatment
- applying hot towels which have been warmed either by soaking in hot water or by warming on a radiator or drying cabinet
- using electrical equipment such as an infra red lamp or thermastatically controlled electrically heated mittens.

Paraffin wax

Paraffin wax is solid and cloudy white in colour when cold. It is heated in a thermostatically controlled wax bath to a working temperature of around 49°C. Paraffin wax treatment is used to ease stiffness in the joints and to improve the texture, colour and condition of the skin. It heats the tissues by enclosing the area with warm wax.

This encourages:
- the skin to perspire
- erythema, to develop
- increased activity in the sebaceous glands
- the pores to open helping the nourishing cream, which has been applied to the hands as part of the treatment, to be absorbed.

Clients who suffer from rheumatism find this treatment helps to relieve pain and stiffness in the joints.

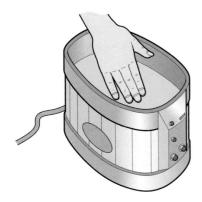

Figure 9.37 Paraffin wax bath

Procedure for paraffin wax treatment

1. The wax must be heated in the wax bath at least 30 minutes before you need to use it. You will have to plan ahead to ensure the wax is properly melted and ready for use.
2. The manicure or pedicure is completed up to and including a brief hand massage. A rich massage cream is applied and gently massaged in to the area.
3. Test the temperature of the wax by first looking at its consistency. Then check the thermostat on the heater and apply wax to the inside of your wrist with a spatula.
4. The clients hand is dipped to just above the wrist five or six times until the hand has a white 'glove' of paraffin wax.

NOTE! There should be a separate wax bath for pedicure. The foot can be treated in exactly the same way as the hand. Alternatively the wax is brushed on to the foot. A good, thick even layer of wax is required.

5. Wrap the hand in tin foil or a plastic bag and cover with a towel.
6. This process is repeated on the other hand.
7. The wax can be left on for up to 20 minutes depending on how much time has been allowed for the manicure. 10 minutes is adequate. Make sure the client is seated comfortably and relaxed.
8. Remove the wax from the first hand. The wax should peel off in one piece and be disposed of.
9. The hand is now in an ideal condition for massage. A full massage of 10 minutes should be given to ensure that the client receives the full benefit of the treatment. Repeat on the other hand.
10. Continue with the application of varnish, taking extra care when wiping over the nails with varnish remover to ensure that there are no traces of wax left on the nails.

Safety precautions

1. Safety checks should be made on the electrical wax bath. The thermostat must be in good working order to ensure that the wax does not overheat.

2. Protect the client's clothing and the area around the wax bath during treatment. The process can be very messy.
3. Do not move the wax whilst it is hot.
4. Dispose of used wax immediately after use.

Oil treatment

The application of good quality warm vegetable oil to the hands can be very beneficial in treating dry cuticles and nails. Almond oil is ideal but because of the quantities required it can prove expensive for use in manicure. Olive oil is most commonly used although it tends to have a distinctive smell.

Procedure for oil treatment

1. Place sufficient oil to cover the fingers of one hand up to the first joint in a small bowl. Place this in a larger bowl of hot water on the manicure table.
2. When the cuticle work is completed on the left hand, the fingers are placed in the bowl of warm oil whilst the right hand is being treated.
3. The left hand is removed and placed on a tissue. It will be necessary to replenish the hot water to warm up the oil for the right hand.
4. The left hand can now be massaged using the oil. Pay particular attention to the cuticles and dry areas of skin. Massage would normally be confined to the hands and wrist.
5. As this is a remedial treatment, the client should be encouraged not to have varnish applied. This allows the nails and cuticles to benefit from the oil soaking in. Any excess can be removed with tissues. If the client prefers, the hands can be wiped over with witch hazel on a pad of cotton wool. The oil treatment can also be used in an oil manicure as a substitute for soaking in soapy water.

Masks

The colour and condition of the hands can be improved by proprietary brand masks which hydrate the skin or which remove unsightly sun spots by gentle bleaching. The masks are applied in the normal way using a masking brush and are removed after 10–15 minutes with warm water.

Exfoliating

Exfoliation is the removal of dead skin using mildly abrasive substances such as ground fruit kernels, oatmeal or salt. Exfoliation treatment for the hands removes dry dead skin scales, ingrained dirt and stains which tend to build up on hard working hands.

- **Chemical exfoliants** are more often used on the feet to treat the build up of hard skin. An alkali breaks down the keratin in the skin, softening it. The product also contains grains which loosen the softened skin. The product must be rinsed off thoroughly to remove any traces of the alkali which would irritate the skin. (Cuticle remover is a similar product which softens the cuticle to aid removal).

Salt or oatmeal rub

Salt is mixed to a paste with water or oil and rubbed on the hands with pads of the fingers using gentle friction movements. Oatmeal mixed and applied in the same way has a similar effect, but is a little more gentle. The salt or oatmeal rub would come before hand massage in the manicure routine.

SELF ASSESSMENT TEST

1. Hot water is essential during the manicure:
   a) to soak the client's nails and cuticles
   b) to wash the towels
   c) to clean the manicure implements
   d) to wipe up any spillages.

2. What is the main reason for using buffing paste when buffing?
   a) to stimulate nail growth
   b) to condition the nails
   c) to improve the colour of the nails
   d) to give the nails a shine.

3. When shaping the nail the emery board should be used:
   a) with a sawing action across the top of the free edge
   b) in one direction towards the centre of the free edge
   c) across the surface of the nail plate
   d) by pulling back the nail wall and filing the free edge to a point.

4. Leuconychia is _____.

5. On which part of the nail is the hyponychium found _____.

6. What is the correct name for the half moon _____.

7. What four words best describe when infection is present _____

   _____ _____ _____.

8. Onychophagy is _____.

9. Pterygium is _____.

10. Give two contraindications to manicure _____ _____.

UNIT 10

Pierce ears

In this unit you will learn about:

- preparing the client for ear piercing
- preparing the ear piercing equipment for use
- how to work hygienically and safely
- working with the restraints of legislation
- how to recognise and advise on contraindications
- piercing the ear lobe
- providing advice in regard to contra-actions and aftercare.

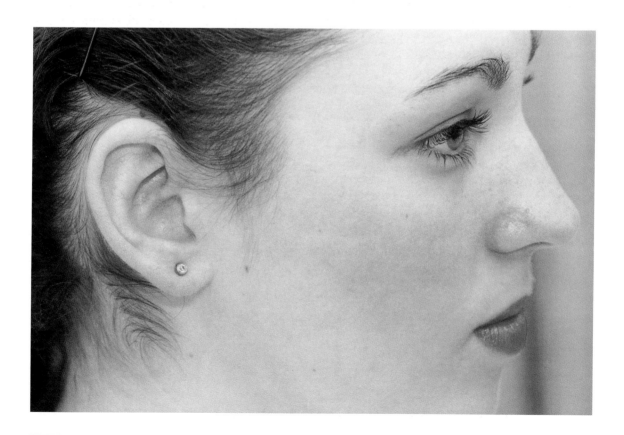

INTRODUCTION

Ear piercing is a quick and inexpensive treatment to perform, but it is profitable. Although it appears as an additional unit to the NVQ qualification and can be performed by receptionists, jewellers, hairdressers as well as therapists, it should not be considered lightly. Ear piercing is an **invasive treatment**, that is to say the skin is broken leaving the wound open to infection. Blood and serum loss may occur. There is a risk of cross infection with the AIDS and Hepatitis B viruses. This has led to stringent control over the performance of this treatment involving the salon registering with the local authority, types of equipment which are disposable, strict hygiene and waste disposal measures.

LEGISLATION

Details of the **Health and Safety at Work Act 1974** and the **Control of Substances Hazardous to Health Regulations 1992** can be found on pages 2 and 4. Special attention should be given to the **Local Government (Miscellaneous Provisions) Act 1982** (further details on page 7).

The Act stipulates that equipment for piercing the skin should be disposable or suitable for sterilisation by an appropriate method such as autoclave or chemical solution. Alternatively, the parts of the equipment that are in contact with the skin during treatment should be disposable. The act also requires waste material from skin piercing to be placed in yellow bin liners and marked as 'contaminated'. The contents have to be collected separately from other waste and incinerated. Any needles or sharps should be placed into a yellow sharps box for special disposal.

HYGIENE

It is essential to maintain high standards of hygiene and professionalism as with all beauty therapy treatments. The following hygiene measures must be carried out for ear piecing:

1. Work surfaces should be wiped down with hot, soapy water or suitable sanitising solution.
2. The ear piecing equipment must meet legal requirements by being disposable or sterile, and is sterilised if appropriate.
3. Wash your hands before and after treatment.
4. Open cuts or wounds on your hands should be covered with a sterile dressing. It is recommended that latex gloves are worn.
5. The area to be treated is checked for contraindications.
6. Treatment is refused politely if there is infection or disease present. You should pay particular attention to ears which have been previously pierced, particularly multiple ear piercing.
7. A non-toxic pen should be used to mark the ear lobe.

EAR PIERCING EQUIPMENT

The ear piecing system should be approved by the Environmental Health Authority under the Local Government Miscellaneous Provisions Act 1982. Stud earrings are more commonly used due to the increased risk of infection from the ring or sleeper type which cannot be inserted in the ear using the gun method. The earrings are sealed in presterilised packs which should only be opened just before use. Where the system includes the use of a gun to pierce, plastic mounting devices are used so the earring remains untouched by hand. The sealed packs often have an expiry date or coloured seal that indicates when the pack should no longer be considered sterile. There is a wide variety of earrings available: different shapes and those with small coloured stones in a variety of colours, as well as the plain round gold type in large or small sizes.

To perform an ear piercing treatment you will need:
1. ear piercing gun
2. studs
3. non-toxic marker pen
4. medical wipes or swabs impregnated with alcohol to cleanse the ears
5. mirror
6. clean cotton wool
7. surgical spirit
8. lined waste bin
9. hair clips
10. disposable latex gloves
11. Aftercare lotion and instruction leaflet.

Contraindications
Conditions preventing treatment
- scar tissue
- bruising
- swelling
- cuts and abrasions
- small ear lobe
- moles and warts
- inflammation
- ear infections
- skin disease or disorder – because of the risk of cross infection, treating someone with an infection could make your insurance invalid.

Conditions requiring medical permission
- Diabetes, due to poor healing ability.
- Epilepsy, the stress and shock involved may induce a fit.
- Circulatory disorders, such as high or low blood pressure.
- Dysfunction of the nervous system, such as lack of sensation in the area.

When a contraindication is apparent the therapist must use tact and diplomacy to inform the client that the service cannot be performed. If medical permission is required the referral should be made without naming the specific condition. The therapist should be able to recognise a possible problem but not to diagnose the condition. Some contraindications may prevent treatment at that time, but can be performed when the condition has receded such as inflammation. Clear yet tactful communication is required to inform the client of the facts without causing embarrassment or anger. This will ensure their return.

Element 10.1

Preparation of the client for ear piercing

The client should be made aware of the procedure, cost, duration, healing time and aftercare before the commencement of the treatment. Therefore, a short but concise consultation is performed which must include the following steps.

1. The area to be treated must be checked for its suitability for piercing. Only the soft tissue of the ear lobe is suitable, as piercing the cartilage leads to overgrowth of the tissue and a condition called **cauliflower ear**. Also infection of cartilage tissue is difficult to treat. Piercing of the nose and other areas of the body are not covered by this unit and special insurance is required to perform these treatments.

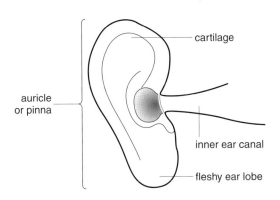

Figure 10.1 The outer ear

2. The age of the client should be asked as you are required by law to gain parental or a guardian's consent in writing before piercing a child under the age of 16. Some salons ask this of clients up to the age of 18. Piercing the ears of a child of preschool age is legal with parental or guardian consent, though some salons may refuse to do this as

part of their own salon policy. It is advisable to write the details of the treatment onto a record card and ask the client (parent or guardian if the client is under 16) to sign to say she has understood and agrees to the treatment being performed.

3. Remember that the client may be nervous so you must appear reassuring and confident in your approach. Provide adequate ventilation and privacy if the client requires it. There should be good lighting and the client should be sat at a height convenient to you. She must be comfortable and able to sit upright with her head level and facing forward.

Element 10.2
Procedure for piercing the ears

1. Discuss with the client the type of earrings required, and their position on the ear.
2. Secure the hair away from the ears with a clip if necessary.
3. Check for contraindications.
4. Wash your hands and put on the disposable latex gloves.
5. With the aid of a mirror, discuss the exact position of the earrings. If there is jewellery already present, it should be removed at this stage.
6. Clean the ear lobes back and front using a separate medical swab for each ear. Allow to dry.
7. Place a small dot on each ear lobe using the non-toxic marker pen to indicate the position of the earrings. Remember the dot should be placed in the fleshy part of the ear and should not be too close to the edge as this may cause tearing if caught accidentally. Ensure the marks are level by using the features of the face as a guide.
8. Check with the client the intended position using a mirror. If incorrect remove with a medical swab, allow to dry and try again. When both you and the client are happy continue the treatment.
9. Load the gun with the earrings according to the manufacturers instructions. Do not touch the earrings and ensure that all disposable guards are in place.
10. Hold the ear to be pierced in your free hand and, with the gun in a horizontal position, place the stem of the stud over the mark made on the ear lobe. Squeeze the trigger gently so the stem is closer to the ear, check the position over the mark and, if correct, squeeze firmly to release the gun and pierce the ear. If not, reposition and repeat.
11. Release the gun by gently pulling downwards while still holding the ear with the other hand.
12. Repeat for the other ear.
13. Show the finished result to the client in the mirror.
14. Instruct the client on aftercare.

15. Clean the gun with surgical spirit on cotton wool and store hygienically for next use.
16. Remove all waste from the area including the gloves and place in the yellow bin for contaminated waste.

AFTERCARE ADVICE

1. Explain to the client that they will initially feel tingling and there may be some redness and slight swelling. If this persists, or any contra-actions arise such as irritation, the

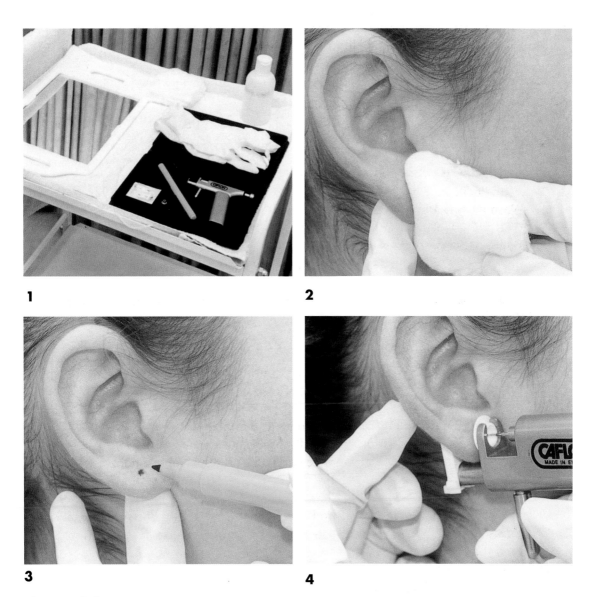

1

2

3

4

Figure 10.2 Steps involved in ear piercing

area becomes sore or begins to weep, the client must inform the salon so that advice can be given and notes made on the client record card.

2. Advice on care of newly pierced ears is to be meticulous in keeping the area clean. Should any contra-actions occur, begin bathing again with salt water or aftercare solution. If the problems continue the client should see a doctor.

3. The earrings should not be removed for 6 weeks. This is to give the ears time to heal properly preventing secondary infection. Premature removal will result in the hole closing up and/or secondary infection.

4. The ears should be bathed twice a day with the aftercare solution or warm salt water.

5. The hands should be washed before the ears are bathed and touching the ears or earrings between bathing should be avoided.

6. After bathing the earrings should be turned to avoid the ear healing on to the stud. To do this hold the back of the earring with one hand whilst turning the stud with the other.

7. Avoid spraying the ears with hairspray or perfume and ensure that shampoo and soap do not accumulate around the stud.

8. After 6 weeks the earrings can be changed. Care should be taken with cheap fashion earrings as they are made of metals that can cause irritation and so should only be worn for short periods of time.

9. If no earrings are worn then the holes are likely to heal over.

10. It is rare for a client to develop a condition called **keloids**, which is the overgrowth of scar tissue. If this does arise, the client should be advised not to have piercing again and, depending on the severity, to remove the earrings and seek medical advice.

11. If allergies occur to the earrings at any time they should be removed immediately and the client instructed to see a doctor if the condition is severe.

It is always advisable to issue a leaflet on aftercare, and also verbally instruct the client on these points.

Activity

Design an aftercare leaflet for ear piercing clients.

SELF ASSESSMENT TEST

1. Which piece of legislation provides the guidelines for ear piercing treatments?
2. Give two examples of these guidelines.
3. Why is only the soft tissue of the earlobe suitable for piercing?
4. List five hygiene precautions to be taken when ear piercing.
5. Why is it important to gain parental or a guardian's consent when piercing a client under the age of 16?
6. Is it illegal to pierce the ears of a child aged two?
7. How often should the ears be cleaned after piercing?
8. How long should the client retain the studs before she can remove them?
9. How would infection of the ear lobe be recognised?
10. What advice would you give to a client if infection were to occur?

Glossary

Acid mantle – the protective film formed on the skin composed of sebum and sweat

Access and egress – terms used in health and safety legislation, refers to the way in and way out of an area

Aftercare – advice to the client regarding things she must do or not do to preserve and maintain the effects of a particular treatment

Confidentiality – privacy given to information which the client has trusted you with

Consultation – a discussion with the client to gain important details and give advice prior to treatment

Contra actions – reactions by the client to the treatment such as excessive erythema

Contra indications – any signs which indicate that a particular treatment should not be carried out, eg infection, open wounds in the area to be treated

COSHH – control of substances hazardous to health regulations, legislation concerned with the safe handling, storage and use of chemicals and other products which are used or sold in the salon

Cosmetics – preparations used to enhance the skin and hair

Couperose skin – redness caused by broken capillaries usually found on the cheeks

Cross infection – infection which passes from one person to another by direct contact or from articles or implements

Dehydrated – lacking in moisture

Desquamation – natural shedding of surface skin cells (stratum corneum)

E-mail – electronic mail which links computers across the world to relay information

Emollient – an ingredient in skin creams which softens

Environmental Health Officer (EHO) – an employee of the local council responsible for checking and implementing standards of health and safety in the work place

Erythema – redness of the skin brought about by physical or chemical stimulus which dilates the capillaries in the skin

Exfoliate – the removal of dead cells from the surface of the skin (epidermis) using either special cosmetics or implements

Fax – facsimile, a means of transmitting paper information using telephone lines

Florid skin – redness caused by a mass of broken capillaries in the skin, usually found on the cheeks and nose

Health and Safety Executive (HSE) – the governing body which regulates the law relating to health and safety

House style – images such as logos or practice which gives a business its individual identity

Hypo-allergenic – cosmetics which are designed for sensitive skin which do not contain perfume or additives

Keloid – overgrown tissue at the site of a scar

Humectant – a substance which attracts water

Keratin – the protein found in skin, hair and nails

Key skills – skills which have been identified as those which are needed to be effective at work and throughout life eg communication

Legislation – the laws which govern the country

Limits of own authority – the extent of your responsibility as determined by your own job description and work place policies

Litigation – legal action such as suing a salon for negligence

Lymph – straw coloured tissue found in the lymphatic system

Medical referral – any condition which requires the client to consult a doctor or other medical practitioner such as a chiropodist

Menopause – the stage in a woman's life when there are major changes in the production of reproductive hormones

Moisturisers – products which help to hydrate the skin by replacing or retaining the water found in the epidermis

Pigmentation – the colour of the skin and hair is determined by the natural pigment called melanin which is produced by cells called melanocytes

Petty cash – a small sum of money available for small items such as coffee or paying the window cleaner etc.

Risk assessment – any risk associated with chemicals or processes used in the salon is assessed usually by the manager and training or guidance given to staff

Sallow skin – yellowish coloured skin associated with an oily skin

Salon services – the treatment available to the client which are printed on the salon price list

Sanitisation – cleansing or washing to an antiseptic level so as to inhibit bacteria

Secondary infection – where an open wound becomes infected

Skin test – products which are known to cause allergic reaction in some people are tested on the skin prior to treatment. A positive result will show as irritation and redness at the site of the test and treatment with that product must not be carried out. A negative result will show that there is no adverse reaction and treatment can continue

Sun Protection Factor (SPF) – a number which gives a guide to the effectiveness of a sun-screening product

Sunscreen – products used on the skin to filter out harmful rays from the sun – UVA and UVB

Technical skills – the practical activities the therapist carries out in treating clients

Terminal hair – course dark hair found on the scalp, under the arms and pubic area

Translucent – allows light to pass through, associated with face powder

Treatment plan – the stages you intend to follow in carrying out a particular treatment or course of treatments to include evaluating the progress and success of the treatment

Vellus hair – fine downy hair found on most areas of the body

Index